Children with Complex
and Continuing Health Needs

Children with Complex and Continuing Health Needs

The Experiences of Children, Families and Care Staff

Jaqui Hewitt-Taylor

Jessica Kingsley Publishers
London and Philadelphia

First published in 2008
by Jessica Kingsley Publishers
116 Pentonville Road
London N1 9JB, UK
and
400 Market Street, Suite 400
Philadelphia, PA 19106, USA

www.jkp.com

Copyright © Jaqui Hewitt-Taylor 2008
Printed digitally since 2009

Library of Congress Cataloging in Publication Data

Hewitt-Taylor, Jaqui.
   Children with complex and continuing health needs : the experiences of children, families and care
staff / Jaqui Hewitt-Taylor.
      p. ; cm.
   Includes bibliographical references and index.
   ISBN 978-1-84310-502-2 (pbk. : alk. paper) 1. Chronically ill children--Care. 2. Children with
disabilities--Care. 3. Chronically ill children--Rehabilitation. 4. Children with disabilities--Rehabilitation.
5. Chronically ill children--Family relationships. 6. Children with disabilities--Family relationships. I.
Title.
   [DNLM: 1. Chronic Disease. 2. Disabled Children. 3. Caregivers. 4. Child. 5. Family Relations. 6.
Long-Term Care. WS 200 H611c 2008]
   RJ380.H49 2008
   618.92--dc22

British Library Cataloguing in Publication Data
A CIP catalogue record for this book is available from the British Library

ISBN 978 1 84310 502 2

To children who have complex and continuing health needs, and their families – especially those who shared their stories for this book.

Also to my two-year-old son, John, who helped me with the typing.

Contents

Preface

This book explores the experiences of children with complex and continuing health needs and their families. Its emphasis is not on the technical or medical aspects of the care or support which they need, but concerns their experiences and worlds. It also includes a section on the perspectives of staff from health and social care settings, so that the views, experiences and opinions of all those who are concerned, day to day, with supporting children and their families can be seen and understood. Chapter 1 provides an overview of the development and support provided for children with complex and continuing health needs and their families. In Chapters 2–10 the experiences of children and their families are discussed. Chapter 11 presents the experiences and views of professionals who support children and their families. Chapter 12 draws together the preceding discussions and links this with the information provided in Chapter 1 in order to highlight important points and to make recommendations for the future.

Children, Young People and their Families

The children, young people and families who have contributed to this book from their experiences are listed below. Some have chosen to have their real names used and some have chosen to use pseudonyms. Three families have also contributed information from their personal websites, which are listed in the References.

Alison's son Peter is five. He has congenital central hypoventilation syndrome and requires assisted ventilation via a tracheostomy when he is asleep.

Cheryl has two children, Zak, aged ten and Sophia, aged seven. Both have congenital central hypoventilation syndrome and require assisted ventilation (using non-invasive positive pressure ventilation (PPV) via a mask) when they are asleep.

Chris and Tracy have three children: Nathan, 16, Joshua, 11, and Mollie, who is two. Mollie was born at 26 weeks' gestation. She lost her twin brother Bailey when they were two weeks old. Mollie has cerebral palsy and some degree of hearing loss. She was discharged home requiring two litres of oxygen per minute, but no longer requires additional oxygen.

Debby and Martin have four children: Nathan, James, Michael and Freya. Michael is six years old and was born at 24 weeks' gestation. During the neo-natal period he required assisted ventilation, had grade three intraventricular haemorrhages, and developed retinopathy of prematurity. He has been left with chronic lung disease of prematurity, has recurrent lower respiratory tract infections, requires supplementary oxygen at night, and is currently being assessed to ascertain the cause of additional sleep-related respiratory problems. Michael has an atrial septal defect and pulmonary stenosis. He also has dysphagia and gastro-oesophageal reflux. As a result of this he has a gastrostomy, through which he receives bolus feed during the day and an overnight feed. Michael has been diagnosed as having autistic spectrum disorder and learning disabilities. Michael's family has consented to the use of information from his website.

Evelyn and Alan have three children, Lauren, Siobhan and Devin. Siobhan is six years old and was born at 28 weeks' gestation. She has cerebral palsy, and in association with this the lower field of her vision is cut. Siobhan had epilepsy, but is now seizure-free, but she has a left club foot that was surgically corrected. Siobhan's family has consented to the use of information from her website.

Helen and John have two sons, William and David. David is 16 and has congenital central hypoventilation syndrome. He requires non-invasive PPV via a nasal cushion when he is asleep. When he was younger, David had seizures, after which he could require resuscitation. His last seizure occurred when he was six years old and he stopped taking anticonvulsants when he was eight.

Jo and Stan have two children, Mitchell (who is Stan's stepson) and Daniel. Mitchell is 14 and Daniel is ten. Mitchell has a neuronal migration disorder, he is blind, has epilepsy, and he has cerebral palsy that affects all his limbs. He has a tracheostomy and a gastrostomy through which he receives his feeds and fluids.

Judy has three children, Simon, Paul and Andrew. Simon is 11 and has cerebral palsy and very severe epilepsy. He is blind and is fed via a gastrostomy.

Mr and Mrs Hethrington have two children, Lucy and Ryan. Lucy is 13 and has Rett syndrome. She also has epilepsy, for which she receives regular anticonvulsant medication and may, in addition, require rectal diazepam or paraldehyde to control her seizures. She also sometimes requires suction and oxygen administration. She is fed via a gastrostomy. Lucy also had craniostenosis at birth.

Rachel and her husband have four daughters, all of whom were born prematurely. Jodie is 11 and was born at 30 weeks' gestation. When she was nine Jodie developed epilepsy and was diagnosed as having neurofibromatosis. Bethany is nine. She was born at 26 weeks' gestation and required assisted ventilation during the neo-natal period. She developed an intraventricular haemorrhage and was later diagnosed as having cerebral palsy, which caused a left hemiplegia. This is now almost completely unnoticeable. Bethany is also asthmatic, and at the age of two she developed epilepsy. From July 2005 she was weaned off anticonvulsants and is now seizure-free. Niamh is six. She was born at 25 weeks' gestation. She required assisted ventilation and developed intraventricular haemorrhages, candida septicaemia, and osteomyelitis during her first four months of life. Niamh has been diagnosed as having spastic diplegic cerebral palsy. She has gross hearing loss in her left ear and has no hearing in her right ear. Emmy is five. She was born at 25 weeks' gestation, required assisted ventilation, had intraventricular haemorrhages during the neo-natal period, and has since been found to have suffered a bleed that affected her brainstem. Emmy has a hypoplastic left lung, chronic lung disease of prematurity, and a severe form of periodic breathing and central apnoea related to her brainstem bleed. She requires oxygen administration and apnoea monitoring overnight. She has severe gastro-oesophageal reflux and has had a fundoplication and a percutaneous endoscopic gastrostomy performed. She was also born with microphthalmos and has a false eye. Rachel has consented to the use of information from her family's website.

Rosemary and Colin have two children, Christian and Hollie. Christian is 21 and Hollie is 18. Christian and Hollie have both been diagnosed as having Kohlschutter syndrome, this being the most likely match to their conditions. Christian has epilepsy, has had a fundoplication and gastrostomy, and he is fed via the gastrostomy. He is very susceptible to chest infections and has developmental delay. Hollie also has epilepsy, poor lung capacity, kyphoses and scoliosis, and developmental delay. She has had a tracheostomy performed to correct sleep apnoea, has had a fundoplication and gastrostomy, and is fed via her gastrostomy. Hollie also has vitiligo and is being investigated for type one neurofibromatosis. Both Hollie and Christian have repeated cases of pneumonia and *Pseudomonas aeruginosa* infections.

Sharon and Trevor have two daughters, Amy and Zoë. Zoë is ten and has cerebral palsy.

Steve and Cheryl have two daughters, Hannah and Philipa. Hannah is three and a half and has Rett syndrome. She has epilepsy, and all her seizures are in her sleep. She has low muscle tone and cannot sit independently.

Val and Tony have two children, Thomas, who is ten, and Catherine, who is six and a half. Catherine has spastic quadriplegia, is blind, and has profound learning difficulties. She is fed via a gastrojejunostomy.

Chapter 1

Children with Complex and Continuing Health Needs

There is an increasing number of children who live with what are described as complex and continuing health needs (DoH 2004). The reasons for this increase include: the number of babies who can now survive premature birth; the lower gestational age at which survival is possible; and biomedical and technical advances which enable infants and children to survive diseases, disorders and accidents that would previously have been incompatible with life.

Although infants and children can survive life-threatening events and situations in ways which were previously unimagined, this can mean that they require medical or technical treatment or intervention for many years, and sometimes for their entire life. In some cases children have needs which are described as 'complex and continuing'. This term indicates that they require what are considered to be complex interventions, and that these interventions are ongoing, rather than necessary to stabilise and treat critical illness. There is no absolute definition of a complex health need (Stalker *et al.* 2003). However, children who are being described as having complex and continuing health needs are often dependent on some form of medical technology, such as assisted ventilation, bi-level positive airways pressure, continuous positive airways pressure, a tracheostomy, feeding via a gastrostomy, intravenous drug administration, peritoneal dialysis or haemodialysis, or require regular and unpredictable drug administration or have difficult-to-manage needs such as frequent seizures.

As well as the difficulty in defining what constitute 'complex and continuing health needs', focusing on children's medical or technical needs often detracts from them being seen as people, rather than as a series of needs or procedures. Landsman (2005) describes the tendency of society to medicalise children who have complex health needs. The result of this approach can be that while ostensibly providing these children and their families with support, the manner in which support is organised and delivered devalues them as people and focuses on tasks, and not the quality of the child's life. A vital aspect of working with children who have complex and continuing health needs, and their families, is to acknowledge these needs, but see beyond them to the person and people involved.

Seeing the Person

Children who have complex and continuing health needs, whatever their specific medical or technical requirements, are, first and foremost, children, with the same rights, needs and aspirations as any other child (DoH 2004). They should not have to face prejudice, bullying or harassment (DoH 2004), and should be treated respectfully (Noyes 2006). Like other people, children with complex and continuing health needs want to be listened to, especially when decisions that affect them are being made (DoH 2004). As Noyes (2006) identifies, children and young people who require long-term assisted ventilation regard being able to make decisions and gain independence as vital aspects of achieving quality of life. However, doing this will be difficult if they are not afforded an opportunity to communicate. In addition, the Human Rights Act 1998 (HMSO 1998) describes how being denied the opportunity to communicate can damage an individual's mental well-being. Treating individuals with respect, facilitating their communication, and involving children in decision-making is therefore vital if they are to enjoy optimum mental as well as physical well-being and achieve a good quality of life.

The extent to which children with complex needs are enabled to form relationships and spend their leisure time as they wish is also important in their quality of life. Action for Leisure and Contact a Family (2003) describes how, like their peers, children and young people with disabilities want to make friends and spend their leisure time with their friends. The organisation highlights that the activities which children and young adults with disabilities are involved in or would like to be involved in are very similar to those which non-disabled children and young adults enjoy engaging in. Noyes (2006) also identifies that children who require long-term medical or technical interventions, like other children, value being able to get out of their homes, have a good social life, and take holidays. This clarifies that children who have disabilities want to form relationships and engage in activities and experiences which are as varied, real and important as those of their peers.

Supporting children who have complex and continuing health needs, and their families, effectively means providing support which will enable children to enjoy the same rights and opportunities as their peers, not simply meet their physical health needs (DoH 2001a, 2004). However, despite this principle being recognised, and there being some examples of good-quality provision and practice, there is evidence that children with complex and continuing health needs continue to find achieving equality difficult. This includes access to play and leisure activities (Action for Leisure and Contact a Family 2003; DoH 2004). Access to leisure activities is often limited, and children who have complex needs often have to use specialist services away from their immediate neighbourhood. This means that they do not have the chance to socialise with their local peer group or develop friendships with children in their area in the way that other children can (DoH 2004). Accessing leisure activities can be further hampered by a lack of accessible transport to areas where facilities exist (DoH 2004). These issues mean that children can miss out on opportunities for enjoyment and fun, and the barriers which society puts in their way can make children feel excluded, and this affects their self-esteem (Noyes 2006).

Education

Children with complex and continuing health needs have the same right to education and learning opportunities as other children. If a child is unable to attend school or college, it not only affects their ability to learn and develop new skills and knowledge but also reduces their chances to socialise with their peers (Berry and Dawkins 2004). It is recommended that, wherever possible, children with additional health or learning needs should be enabled to learn in a mainstream education environment unless their parents or guardians choose otherwise or this is 'incompatible with the efficient education of other children' and there are no 'reasonable steps' which the school and local education authority can take to prevent that incompatibility (OFSTED 2004). In addition, the Disability Discrimination Act 2005 (HMSO 2005) places duties on schools not to treat disabled pupils less favourably than others and to make 'reasonable adjustments' to ensure that they are not disadvantaged (OFSTED 2004).

Despite these moves at policy level, the inclusion of all children in mainstream education is not always achieved in practice. Berry and Dawkins (2004) identify that children who have health-related needs (such as tube feeding or the administration of medication during school hours) may be excluded from mainstream education because there are not enough staff who can perform these tasks, rather than because the child is unable to engage in education in a mainstream environment. A lack of suitable transport may also preclude some children from attending the best school for them. Overall, Berry and Dawkins (2004) found that children with complex and continuing health needs may have little or no choice over the school which they attend. They may also be excluded from aspects of the curriculum or have enforced absence from school because of a lack of staff who can meet their day-to-day needs, rather than because of ill health.

As well as having an adverse effect on children, problems in enabling children to access education can affect their families and carers, who often have to be available during school hours in case their child is sent home, and may have to attend school themselves to assist with medical procedures (Berry and Dawkins 2004). A common cause of the problems associated with providing children who have complex and continuing health needs with equal education opportunities is a lack of clarity as to which service is responsible for the child's needs and a failure of heath and education authorities to work together to meet the health needs of children while they are at school (Berry and Dawkins 2004).

Once children are ready to access further education, they and their families may face additional challenges. There is some evidence that further education colleges can experience problems in supporting students who use specialist communication systems or those who have highly specialised but relatively low-incidence needs. In addition, appropriate specialist support may not exist, organising transport, escorts and assistance for personal care may be problematic, and where services have cost implications reaching an agreement over funding them may be difficult and protracted (Millar and Aitken 2005).

Enabling Children to Live at Home

The increasing numbers of children with complex and continuing health needs, and recognition of the importance of meeting all their needs and not just treating their physical problems has required service providers to rethink how and where they are supported. The type of interventions which many children need would traditionally mean that they underwent long-term, sometimes lifelong, hospitalisation. Where the interventions included assisted ventilation it would mean that their care was provided in an intensive care unit setting. However, this situation is now generally seen as inappropriate.

The *National Service Framework for Paediatric Intensive Care* (DoH 1998) identified that intensive care units are not an appropriate place to care for children who require long-term assisted ventilation but are otherwise medically stable. The majority of children in intensive care units are acutely critically ill, and a child who is housed on an intensive care unit will almost inevitably be exposed to sights, sounds and disturbances in their day which are not beneficial to them developmentally or emotionally. The children around them will often appear unresponsive, and will not able to play and interact with other children. Their sleep is likely to be disturbed by lighting and noise which is necessary for the stabilisation and care of acutely critically ill children, but disruptive to the development of normal sleep patterns. At best their parents will usually have to reside in a room within the critical care complex, but away from the intensive care unit, from where they cannot maintain the natural contact that they would have in the family home. The child will usually be confined to one room or bed space, with visits from family and friends, and trips out will be specifically organised. If a single room is not available, the child will have extremely limited privacy. Contact with their siblings and extended family will therefore be very different from what it would be if they were at home. Their mobility will be constrained by the environment, if not by their physical needs, and their ability to access education will be limited by their location.

Despite staff on paediatric intensive care units appreciating the importance of developmental experiences and facilitating the growth of normal family relationships, when the competing demands on them include carrying out life-saving and preserving interventions, providing developmental experiences for a child who is medically stable is likely to hold lower priority. This does not mean that staff do not value or appreciate the needs of children who require long-term interventions. In the real world of healthcare, where the resources, including staff, are finite and the demand is infinite, priorities must be decided. In intensive care, critical illness management and sustaining life is usually the priority, and intensive care units are not designed to provide long-term care. It is therefore almost inevitable that children who are cared for long term in an intensive care unit will be exposed to over- or understimulation and they will lack normal developmental experiences (Boosfeld and O'Toole 2000).

Even outside the intensive care environment, an acute hospital setting is an inappropriate place for children to grow up. In children's wards, although the other children are not as acutely or critically ill as those on intensive care units, they will not provide the type of peer relationships which children would usually experience. Children will not be exposed to the same interactions with adults as they would be at home, and it will be difficult for them to develop awareness of social norms. Parents who care for their child in hospital must effectively 'parent in public' and have very limited privacy, both for establishing a relationship with their child and for conducting their own relationships. For staff who have many demands on their time, facilitating normal developmental experiences for children who require long-term care cannot always be their priority and the range of staff who care for children in a hospital setting makes establishing consistent practices problematic.

It is often difficult for families to maintain the kind of input into their child's care that they want to when care is provided in the hospital environment. Travelling to hospital, and often to a hospital which is distant from their home if specialist care is needed, means that visiting is not easy. Although accommodation for parents is available in most hospitals, this often means either a bed beside their child's bed, with limited additional facilities, or a shared room some distance from the ward. If the family has other children, the parent's contact with them and the child's contact with their siblings will be disrupted when one child is hospitalised long term. Input from the extended family and family friends will also be disrupted. This may include relatives having to travel some distance to visit, restrictions on visiting so that the child cannot see large family groups together, and parents having relatively little opportunity for social support and maintaining relationships with friends and family.

The increase in the number of children requiring complex technological or medical interventions has been accompanied by a recognition that, wherever possible, all children should be cared for at home, as their emotional, psychological, developmental, educational and social needs are generally better met in this environment (Balling and McCubbin 2001; Neufeld, Query and Drummond 2001). Clearly, if children are to achieve equality of opportunity for play and other leisure activities, development of peer relationships, and education, a hospital environment is an inappropriate one for them. Apart from the social and developmental aspects of care, there is also some evidence that children with complex and continuing health needs have better physical health when they are cared for at home rather than in hospital (Appierto et al. 2002).

From the point of view of ownership of their child and empowerment, Taylor (2000) suggests that children and their families are generally provided with better information about their child's needs when their care is provided outside the hospital environment. In hospital, the power ratio is tipped in favour of healthcare staff, and parents are visitors in an unfamiliar environment. This situation is somewhat reversed in the family home, where healthcare staff are the visitors and have a greater obligation to respect the family's rules, values, norms and ownership of their child.

Obstacles to Home Care

Despite the recognition that living at home is usually the ideal option for children and their families, setting up the services which will enable children with complex and continuing health needs to be discharged from hospital is often a problematic and protracted process (DoH 2004). In addition, although the initial setting up of the necessary services may be difficult to effect, it is equally important to ensure that the ongoing support that these children and their families need is in place (Brazier 2006; DoH 2004).

Considerable planning and co-operation between services is needed for children with complex and continuing health needs to be discharged home, including ongoing liaison between hospital and community staff, and collaboration between nursing staff, medical staff, physiotherapists, occupational therapists, education services, social services and equipment suppliers. Despite good intentions, in a busy work environment where many competing demands exist, it may be difficult to achieve the degree of intra- and inter-disciplinary communication and collaboration between hospital and primary care that is needed to achieve this.

Facilitating home care provision also requires staff who are able to support children and their families during the discharge process and after following their discharge home. Recruiting and retaining staff to fulfil such roles is often difficult, particularly as the demand for their services is unpredictable (Hewitt-Taylor 2005). When it becomes clear that a child will require long-term intervention and home care is the goal, a team of staff must be found who can assist in meeting the child's needs. Frequently, this includes services which span both health and social care provision. From the healthcare perspective, neither the National Health Service nor a primary care trust may be expected to have a bank of staff employed awaiting such needs to arise. This means that families must often wait while decisions are made about how and by whom support will be provided, and, in many cases, whilst staff are recruited and trained to assist them.

It has been suggested that caring for children with complex and continuing health needs in an acute hospital setting is an inappropriate use of resources (Boosfeld and O'Toole 2000) and that home care is the more cost-effective option for the National Health Service. However, the initial set-up costs of home care are often high, despite this being the most cost-effective option over time. Once a child is discharged from hospital, the primary care trust in the child's home area, rather than a specialist hospital or acute trust is generally required to provide equipment, consumables, and nursing support to meet their health needs (Glendinning and Kirk 2000). Prescribing costs shift to the primary care trust and local authorities have to provide support in the child's home and school. This may mean that negotiations over funding must be resolved before home care can be achieved (Glendinning and Kirk 2000).

Where children with complex and continuing health needs are cared for in the family home, as well as staff having to be trained to assist them, their parents often have to develop new skills and knowledge, for which they usually require teaching and the opportunity to develop confidence (Boosfeld and O'Toole 2000; DoH 2004). Again, achieving this may take some time and requires staff to be available to work with and support parents in developing their skills. In addition, families must be able, practically and emotionally, to take on the workload of supporting their child's needs, albeit with support from other agencies.

The cost, in financial and emotional terms, for a family to care for a child at home is potentially high and may be a burden which the family is unable to bear, despite the advantages of home care and despite them wanting to look after their child at home. When decisions are made about where and by who a child with complex and continuing health needs is cared for, who will benefit and whose benefit is the most important must be considered. For example, the benefit to the child, their siblings, or the parents must all be taken into account. Although the child's well-being is paramount, every child's well-being, including that of siblings, must be included in the decision-making process. This does not mean that home care is not desirable or, in principle, the 'best' option. However, what is best will not be the same for every child or family. For some children and families, caring for their child at home is not the best option. Where this decision is reached, the family should be offered support to enable them to cope with the difficult decisions that has been made and to continue to have meaningful input into their child's life (Parker et al. 2006).

Caring for a Child at Home

Where a child is cared for at home, the parents theoretically have greater control than they would in a hospital or residential setting because they are on their own territory. However, there are still many factors which disrupt their lives and over which they do not have complete control (Wang and Barnard 2004). The number of individuals and services involved in supporting them can leave them feeling overwhelmed by visits from a range of professionals and can impinge on their privacy and everyday activities (Glendinning and Kirk 2000; Wang and Barnard 2004). Despite being capable of and willing to care for their child, many parents require assistance to manage their child's care on a day-to-day basis. Providing staff to assist families has advantages, and is often essential to enable them to care for their child at home. However, it intrudes on a family whose life-style is already disrupted (Valkenier, Hayes and McElheran 2002). The provision of home-based support requires negotiation of roles and the responsibilities related to medical procedures. It also, and perhaps more problematically, requires negotiation of non-medical aspects of care, such as child-rearing expectations, relationships between carers and the family, and how the family home will be used by care staff (O'Brien and Wegner 2002). Although parents may not need to 'parent in public' in the way that they would in hospital, where healthcare staff are frequent visitors in the family home, and especially in situations where 24-hour input is needed, family relationships are conducted in the presence of others. Parents' childcare practices may be subject to comments and advice unrelated to their medical or technical needs which would not be made if their child did not require staff to be present in the family home. Disruption to family life applies not only to visitors to the home, but also to appointments which children and their families have to attend (DoH 2004). This can add to a situation in which, despite having to provide care for their child 24 hours a day, parents have very little time to do basic household tasks and spend time alone with their children.

Obtaining equipment and supplies can be another time-consuming and stressful aspect of caring for a child who has complex and continuing health needs (DoH 2004). Parents may have to travel to collect supplies, which may be difficult to transport, or the delivery of essential items may be unreliable and mean that parents have to travel at short notice to obtain them. Given the problems inherent in organising even short journeys from the home when a child with complex and continuing health needs is part of the equation this can be a major, inconvenient and costly undertaking for families. Where a child's condition is unpredictable, making an accurate estimate of what will be needed is often impossible, something that suppliers may not understand. This may mean parents having to repeatedly negotiate their needs, and to make additional journeys to collect items that they require.

Parents whose children have complex and continuing health needs have to develop a range of practical skills and knowledge about their child's condition. They also have to acquire complex decision-making skills about the intricacies of their child's condition and the fine-tuning of the interventions and care that the child needs. Although parents develop skills and knowledge that make them uniquely able to care for their child, and very specialist parents, this can also significantly alter the meaning of parenting for them and their expected roles as parents (Kirk, Glendinning and Callery 2005). The practicalities of care provision are often the focus of teaching and support for parents, but Kirk *et al.* (2005) identify that caring for a child who has complex and continuing health needs also has a substantial emotional element. This includes the potential conflict in the nurturing and protecting role, which parents expect to take on, and carrying out clinical procedures, which would, in a hospital setting, be carried out by professionals.

There is also a physically relentless parents' workload. Although they are frequently providing care and interventions that would usually be the remit of professional staff, families have no time off-duty. Wang and Barnard (2004) describe the parents' need to devote extraordinary attention to meeting their child's needs. As well as constant demands on their time during the day, they often have disturbed sleep because of the need to monitor their child or provide input at night long after they would expect a child to be sleeping through the night. This, and the organisational issues involved in ensuring adequate support for their child, alongside all the other aspects of family life which parents have to deal with means that each day can feel like 'one endless battle' (Contact a Family 2004). The level of responsibility which parents take on, and its duration, as well as the physical workload, is often extremely high and stressful (Carnevale *et al.* 2006). Unsurprisingly, given these physical and emotional demands, parents whose children have complex and continuing needs often experience health problems associated with their role as a carer, including physical problems such as back and joint pain from lifting and handling, or problems with their mental health and well-being (Contact a Family 2004).

Despite this, many parents report that their children enrich their lives and provide them with significant rewards, which they could not imagine living without (Carnevale *et al.* 2006). This conflict of emotional and physical stress with enrichment and pleasure is one which parents learn to live with and which service providers need to appreciate in order to provide effective support.

Effects on the Family

Although home care is generally considered to be in the best interests of the child and to disrupt family functioning less than long-term hospitalisation, it can still present challenges to family functioning. A child with complex and continuing health needs living at home may mean that the family home needs to be adapted, or that the family has to move to a more suitable property or location. It will also have an effect on the lifestyle and roles of both parents and siblings. Although Appierto *et al.* (2002) identify care at home as the most cost-effective option for children with complex and continuing health needs, it may shift some of the financial burden from the National Health Service to the family (O'Brien and Wegner 2002). Although the cost of home care may ostensibly be met by the National Health Service and social services, many incidental expenses are met by the family. It is estimated that the cost of bringing up a disabled child is three times higher than bringing up a child who is not disabled (DoH 2004). In addition, the parents' ability to remain in employment, and the type of employment that they can engage in, is likely to be affected by having a child with disabilities, making their income lower while their outgoings are increased (DoH 2004). Only 16 per cent of mothers with disabled children are employed, compared with 61 per cent of other mothers (Brazier 2006). The reasons for this include a lack of childcare to enable them to work, the need for them to take time off work for hospital visits and appointments, and a lack of understanding and flexibility from employers (Contact a Family 2004). Although parents may receive state benefits for caring for their child, in many cases this will not be equivalent to their previous salary, and parents often report difficulty in finding out about and claiming the benefits that they are entitled to (DoH 2004).

As well as the financial aspects of loss of employment, changes in employment status may affect the parents' sense of identity, for example, if their career pathway is unexpectedly terminated. Changes in employment may also alter their social interactions or opportunities. Parents may also find that they lose common ground or experience with friends, that they lose contact with friends or family, or that friends and relatives lose contact with them for a variety of reasons. Meeting friends can be problematic for parents because of the amount of things that they have to juggle related to their child's care. When families go out with their child, they often experience negative or offensive reactions from others and feel that their child's life is devalued (Carnevale *et al.* 2006). This can discourage them from going out with their child, and create a degree of social isolation. Thus, families may find that existing social support networks decrease at a time when their need for support is high. Relationships between parents may also alter or become a source of stress when their child has complex and continuing health needs, and although some parents report that caring for their child brings them closer together, for others it can cause problems in their relationship (Contact a Family 2004).

Going out with a child who has complex and continuing health needs may be very difficult to organise, because of the equipment that is needed and the transport facilities which are available. This means that day-to-day events and taking the family out can become a major undertaking for parents, and events which other families might take for granted, such as taking siblings to and from out of school activities, requires considerable planning. If a family wants to go on holiday, it often requires many months of planning and organisation. Travelling abroad may be so difficult and costly that families do not attempt it (Glendinning and Kirk 2000).

Siblings

Having a brother or sister who has complex or continuing health needs may affect siblings. Taylor, Fuggle and Charman (2001) identify many factors that contribute to how siblings adjust to their brother's or sister's illness, including their attitude towards the illness, their own adjustment to it, their own self-esteem, and feelings of social support, including their mother's awareness of their feelings. Sharpe and Rossiter (2002) suggest that siblings have greater problems if their brother or sister requires daily treatment. Taylor *et al.* (2001) also found that the effects which a child's illness has on overall family functioning, the degree of emotional distress that their mother experiences, and siblings' relationships with adults other than their parents affect their coping and adjustment to their brother's or sister's needs, and the alterations that this causes to their lifestyle.

As well as the effects which a child having complex and continuing health needs may have on their siblings, concerns about this can add to parental stress (Taylor *et al.* 2001). Although a child having complex needs may have adverse effects on their siblings, this is not inevitable (Taylor *et al.* 2001). A child having complex and continuing health needs is likely to have some effect on all members of their family, including siblings, and although this needs to be remembered, the positive as well as negative influences of their experiences should also be considered.

Short-break Services

In addition to providing day-to-day support for families with a child who has complex and continuing health needs, providing parents with short-break services so that they can have some time off from their role as carers is important (DoH 2004; MacDonald and Callery 2004; Neufeld *et al.* 2001; Olsen and Maslin-Prothero 2001). However, short-break services or the opportunity to have a break from caring is one of parents' most frequently reported unmet needs (DoH 2004). There are often waiting lists for short-break care, and children with complex and continuing health needs and those with profound disabilities are more likely to have to wait for such services than others (Shared Care Network 2003). Where short-break services are available they usually have to be planned in advance, and accessing provision at short notice, for example if a parent becomes unwell is often very difficult (Olsen and Maslin-Prothero 2001). In addition, the best way of providing short-break services for families varies. For example, MacDonald and Callery (2004) found notable differences between parents' and carers' views on the best way of providing short breaks. Service provision should, therefore, allow for flexibility according to the needs and preferences of children and their families.

Transition to Adult Services

When children who have complex and continuing health needs reach the time of transition to adulthood both they and their families may be presented with specific challenges in relation to support because the providers of their services change. Perhaps poor co-ordination between the relevant agencies and inadequate healthcare plans at the time of transfer make planning service provision and accessing adult services difficult (DoH 2001a). Local agencies are required to have a system of person-centred planning for all young people moving from children's to adult's services and to provide effective links between children's and adult's services in both health and social care (DoH 2001a). However, the *National Service*

Framework for Children, Young People and Maternity Services (DoH 2004) identifies that transition planning to adult services is still often unsatisfactory, with a lack of co-ordination between services and little involvement of the young person.

Supporting Experts

The families of children with complex and continuing health needs, and the children themselves, soon become experts in their care. They are often far more knowledgeable about the practicalities and intricacies of care and the underlying disease processes than many healthcare professionals, and are frequently involved in teaching professionals about these (DoH 2001b). Glendinning and Kirk (2000) identify that the families of such children regularly perform procedures, such as changing tracheostomy tubes and initiating and supervising assisted ventilation, which are outside the knowledge or experience of some healthcare staff. Parents also become experts in monitoring their child's condition and are often able to detect changes earlier than professionals, using intuition and knowledge of their child rather than measurable parameters as their guides (Kirk *et al.* 2005). Although this is necessary and desirable, and parents' knowledge of their child's condition and care needs adds to their empowerment, caring for an expert family may also be daunting for professionals. Glendinning and Kirk (2000) found that some professionals feel threatened by expert parents and some parents felt that professionals avoided them for this reason. A challenge for professionals is to work in partnership with families: sharing knowledge, skills and resources. Donaldson (2003) suggests that achieving this type of partnership working requires changes in attitudes and modes of interaction by both healthcare professionals and service users. However, this balance is not easy to achieve and requires consistent negotiation, effort and honesty on both sides.

Summary

There is likely to be an ever-increasing number of children and young people who require long-term medical and technical interventions. The care of children with complex and continuing healthcare needs requires those supporting them to be aware of their physical needs, but also their psychosocial and developmental needs, and the needs of the family as a whole. The most important part of providing support is to see the child first and foremost as an individual, and not a child with complex and continuing health needs. It is clearly vital that the staff who provide input related to the child's medical and technical needs are competent in these aspects of care provision. However, the real challenge and the skill of supporting children and their families lies in the ability to understand their world, or the part of it which is shared, to provide humanistic, not just technically competent care, and, respectfully, to seek to enhance their quality of life. This means incorporating knowledge of treatment and interventions into the provision of support which, first and foremost, considers the child and family to have social, developmental, educational, emotional and spiritual, as well as technical and medical, needs.

Chapter 2

Being a Child or Young Person with Complex Needs

Children and young people who have complex and continuing health needs should be seen first and foremost as individuals and as children or young people with the same needs and rights as any other person. However, some parents have reported that the person who is their child can become lost in concerns about their medical or technical needs, and their opportunities may be reduced because of this. For example, Jo has discovered that, in certain situations, activities that Mitchell would enjoy have become impossible because he has a tracheostomy, not because a tracheostomy is incompatible with the activities, but because some services 'don't take traches'. Situations such as this, combined with their needs, mean that children and young people with complex and continuing health needs often have to make a great deal more effort than other children or young people to be afforded opportunities and to achieve their potential. This chapter discusses some of the areas in which children should be enabled to enjoy the same opportunities as their peers, and presents some of the barriers to this being achieved.

Communication

Communicating with other people is an everyday part of life. However, some children have to make a great deal more effort than others to communicate, not necessarily because their understanding is impaired, but because making themselves understood is a problem. This may be because they have difficulty in speaking and have to make an additional effort and expend greater energy in learning to speak and co-ordinating their speech. In some cases, children have the potential to learn to speak, but their ability to achieve this is diminished because their abilities are not recognised, their efforts are not rewarded, and they are not afforded an opportunity to learn to speak. For example, Rosemary recalls that it was not until he went to college at the age of 19 that Christian's abilities were recognised and as a result, 'Christian is just starting to make sounds and learning how to project his voice'. Rosemary also describes trying to procure a speaking valve for Hollie's tracheostomy: 'To give her the opportunity to see if she could use it, but the attitude you receive is: "Will she speak?" No. "Did she speak before the tracheostomy?" No. "So what's the point of her having a speaking valve?" The point is *opportunity*, to be given the benefit of choice. To be given the right to develop skills to improve her life through additional methods of communication.' Given that Hollie's brother has only recently had the opportunity to learn to speak, at a college where Hollie hopes soon to enrol, a disinclination to afford her this opportunity seems particularly unfortunate.

The provision of specialist services to assist children to learn to speak may also be lacking. Rosemary has found the task of trying to find a speech and language therapist who works with children and young people with learning disabilities almost impossible to achieve. She explains that, although health authorities have a duty of care which includes providing speech and language therapy, the policies that are in place related to this are not always followed because of a lack of speech and language therapists who have received training to enable them to work with people who have learning disabilities. She describes how this appears to be a result of divisions between services, which often makes it difficult for individuals to specialise in speech and language therapy and learning disabilities.

The effort which individuals may need to make to speak can be increased by having to deal with negative responses to their efforts. Rosemary describes how, when Christian attempts to speak to his carers, in some cases 'if he is not completely ignored, the most inventive response they can think of is: "Oh yes, what else?" Even worse, they mimic his voice.' This disinclination to take seriously children's attempts at speaking, or the idea that the person might wish to or be able to communicate, can clearly discourage them from making the effort to communicate, which in turn reinforces the belief that they cannot do so. As Rosemary comments this situation means that the child or young person becomes 'a self-fulfilling prophecy'.

Where a child uses alternative means of communication, such as signing or a communication aid, learning to use and using these requires additional time and effort on their part. It also often means that they have to make considerable effort to engage others in communicating with them and rely on individuals being sufficiently motivated to learn their way of communicating. This becomes even more of a challenge where children communicate through very subtle non-verbal signs. Rosemary explains that 'Hollie is unable to make any sounds now that she has her tracheostomy, but she speaks with her eyes. When talking to Hollie or Christian it is important to watch body language: their eyes, their facial expressions, even their eyebrows, and their hands, and yes both hands as well as the fingers and thumbs. Listen out for even the smallest of sounds, or the difference of breaths. With experience you may be able to notice that in fact, they are communicating all the time.' Rosemary explains that the common misconception that a person who cannot communicate using well-recognised forms of communication does not have thoughts, ideas or feelings which they wish to communicate is highly misleading, and rather 'we have to learn how to speak their language'.

In some instances, however, learning a person's language is very difficult. Jo describes how her entire relationship with Mitchell is based on intuitive knowledge, nuances of movement, and demeanour: 'You are talking about instincts, and it's amazing how that instinct develops…what actually goes on in the relationship between a mum and a child who doesn't talk. The whole relationship is based on a different level, made up of completely different skills. There's something between Mitchell and I that, spiritually, we work on a sixth-sense level.' What is clear is that, despite the complexity of this, Mitchell does communicate. The challenge is for those who are involved with him to find ways, including using Jo as an interpreter, to communicate with Mitchell.

In many cases, parents report that their child's difficulty in speaking or their disability is mistaken for an inability to understand, for example, children being excluded from conversations, or talked over, even when these directly concern them. Sharon explains how many people 'won't actually talk to Zoë. But she understands. So I say "Talk to her, I will interpret her answers if you don't understand, but talk to her, not me. I don't know what she's feeling, what she's thinking at the moment."' Rosemary also describes how, in healthcare settings, it is extremely rare for Hollie and Christian to be included in information giving and how 'they are talked over'. This can mean that as well as the additional effort that children have to make to communicate, they must bear the frustration and anger which can result from being excluded from conversations which concern them, which occur in their presence, and which they can understand.

Even when a child's level of understanding is not clear, giving them opportunities to understand and communicating in a way which includes them and gives them a chance to be involved is essential. As Cheryl explains: 'The research doctor says that Hannah has very little understanding, and I don't know if she does, sometimes I think she does understand things. Sometimes I think she doesn't. We've been told her understanding is very very limited. But she does sometimes just laugh in exactly the right places. It's a strange thing not knowing what someone understands. Sometimes people will talk about her in the room and I think I wonder what she's thinking. We feel it is very important to speak and approach Hannah as if she understands fully.' As Steve says, 'she is a human being and she may feel things emotionally in the same way we do'.

Play and Enjoyment

Children with complex and continuing health needs have the same right to pleasure, play and developmental opportunities, and to choose the activities which they want to engage in as other children. Steve and Cheryl stress how important it is that, like any other child, Hannah should 'have the opportunity to have fun', for no other reason than enjoyment. Jo also describes the importance of Mitchell having the chance to simply enjoy himself. She describes a recent occasion when he went with Stan and some other lads to play football. Although Mitchell could not join in the activity itself, he loved the atmosphere and being a part of the social interactions. Children being able to choose the activities which they enjoy is also important. As Sharon describes, like any other child, 'Zoë knows the things she wants to do, so she goes to swimming lessons, she goes to Brownies and stuff.'

However, in many cases it is much harder for children who have complex and continuing health needs to experience opportunities for play, recreation and enjoyable activities which their peers take for granted. This may be because their physical needs preclude some activities. For example, children being unable to eat may alter their opportunities for pleasure. Jo explains that when Mitchell had a gastrostomy performed and could no longer eat it removed, albeit necessarily, one of the pleasures in his life. A child's needs may also make engaging in play harder or more physically tiring for them than for other children. In other instances, children may be able to engage in the same play activities as their peers, but need to be cautious of over-exertion. Alison describes how 'Peter might be tearing around the playground like everyone else, but because his respiratory control isn't the same as anyone else's, he might sometimes need to be told to slow down.' Sometimes though, as described in more detail in Chapter 10, children's ability to enjoy themselves is restricted by a lack of facilities which cater for their needs. Sharon illustrates this point: 'I can't take Zoë to soft play because she can't walk round it, and they're not built for adults to get round so I might be able to get her halfway up and then she's stuck because I can't go and retrieve her.'

Many children have needs that mean that spontaneity is difficult for them. As Sharon describes, Zoë's needs affect her ability to play spontaneously: 'If Zoë wants to go out and play in the garden, I have to mat all the patio, because she can't walk and she needs to be safe out there, and it takes so long to set up. Other kids are in and out and in and out, but for her you have to actually plan things in advance.' Children with complex and continuing health needs therefore often depend on others being available to set up and supervise their play or enjoyment, creating or facilitating opportunities for them, seeing this as a priority, and understanding the importance of enjoyment, play and stimulation in their lives. Rosemary explains that achieving this for Hollie and Christian on a day-to-day basis can be problematic: 'What they [many of the carers who work with Hollie and Christian] can't understand is that every single thing Hollie or Christian does is something they store in their memory. I always think, at the end of every day: What has Hollie done today? What has Christian done today? What have they done that has enriched their lives? What have they learnt today, that they did not know yesterday? And if all they have done is be put in front of the automatic babysitter, called the TV, or gone up and down the road for a walk to the post box, what are they going to dream about?'

Education

The issues involved in children accessing the best education opportunities for them are described in Chapter 9. However, even when a child is able to access high-quality education, they may often have to make a much greater effort to achieve what their peers achieve at school or college. This may be because of health-related issues, including missing school because of ill health, ill health affecting their ability to concentrate on learning, and health-related appointments causing them to miss school and having to find the time to catch up with their peers. Cheryl explains that Zak struggles to keep up with his peers at school because of 'all the little things, like he misses so much school for hospital appointments'.

Learning can also pose a greater workload for some children because the way in which they learn requires more effort than the way in which other children learn. Evelyn describes how 'I am really proud of Siobhan. She just tries so hard. She has to try so much harder than other children, and she achieves so much. She doesn't always achieve everything but she tries so hard and she gets so tired from just having to use so much more energy.' Although Siobhan does extremely well at school, Evelyn reports that she has to continue with her schoolwork during the holidays to prevent her losing the progress and achievements of the previous term. This means that, as Evelyn explains, 'she doesn't really get a summer holiday'.

In some instances, it seems that people failing to see the child or young person as an individual who can make choices means that their intellectual ability, achievements and potential to achieve are assessed inaccurately. Rosemary describes how the assumption is: 'If you don't do what I expect, I assume you can't cognitively do it.' To illustrate this point Rosemary recalls, 'When computers began to be used in schools, the staff tried to get Christian to use a computer. To start the program, a green frog appeared on the screen and Christian had to hit a switch which made a gun appear and shoot the frog. The screen turned red, and then the programme started. Christian did not want to kill the frog, so he was labelled as unable to use the switch or understand what was required of him. It was decided that he was intellectually unable to do it. I said: "No, Christian does not want to kill the frog."' An alternative scenario was produced for Christian: the screen showed two soldiers, and by using the switch, Christian would fire a shot, killing the soldiers. However, as Rosemary notes, 'Killing is not something he does. So he failed his assessment because it was assumed he couldn't do it. But, he could do it, he just didn't choose to kill people. No one thinks about whether or not he wants to do something.'

Privacy

There are many barriers to children with complex and continuing health needs having the degree of privacy which their peers enjoy. As well as needing assistance with physical care, they may need an adult to be present during their play and leisure activities and other social interactions. As David and Helen explain, despite David needing one-to-one support at school, 'his one-to-one could drive him mad being there all the time'. In some cases children need to have an adult present when they are asleep, and although this may not intrude on social or peer interactions in the way that a third party being present with them during the day does, it limits their privacy. David requires assisted ventilation overnight, and has carers to supervise this. Helen describes how, to maximise his privacy and to provide the carers with facilities the family has a separate sitting room beside David's room for staff to use at night.

As well as physical privacy, children may wish to keep information about their health needs private, but requiring support may make this difficult. For example, David likes to keep his medical condition private, and if the family has visitors, he prefers not to have a carer during that time so that their presence does not require explanation. Although David's family can manage this, because of the need for some disclosure about their medical condition for safety purposes, children often have to rely on others to maintain their privacy of information, and this may not always be respected. Helen describes how 'David loves sport, and he wanted to do tennis. So I went to the local tennis club, explained about David, and that was fine. But then on the first day I took him and the coach said, in front of all the other children and mothers: "Oh, I've thought about this, and David and his medical condition, and I don't want to take the responsibility, so I'd rather you stay." ...David was just mortified. She could have thought about it and called me to one side and had a quiet word or phoned me.' This type of experience means that, as Helen explains, children and their families may have to make decisions about how to balance their safety and their right to privacy, which other children may not need to make.

Social Opportunities

Like all children, children who have complex and continuing health needs should have the chance to socialise and interact with their peers. However, in some cases, their physical needs mean that they cannot participate fully in all social situations no matter how much effort is made. For example, Rachel is aware that Emmy cannot view certain films because she has one false eye: 'You need both eyes for 3D: she won't be able to see 3D films. She won't be able to go to the cinema with her friends and watch 3D movies.' Children who have altered feeding patterns or have difficulty eating may also have difficulties participating fully in or enjoying social events such as parties, meals out and celebrations, or simply joining in mealtimes with their peers. Rosemary highlights issues around mealtimes for children who are fed using a gastrostomy, and contrasts the extent to which policies and practices at different schools enable children to be included with their peers. At Hollie's school the children who require gastrostomy feeding are fed in a room away from the other children. In contrast, at the further education college where Christian attends, all the students spend their mealtimes together, with those requiring gastrostomy feeding having their meal alongside the others. As Rosemary comments, 'this is called inclusion!'

Although their physical needs may alter a child's social opportunities, the facilities for children with complex and continuing health needs to engage in social situations and interact with other children are often a significant limitation to their social lives. Judy explains how Simon goes to one of the few groups which integrates children with complex needs with others: Chickenshed, an amateur dramatics company. However, his experience there illustrates how difficult full integration can be, even where organisations make considerable effort. As Judy recounts: 'They didn't really know how to cope with a child with his level of complexity. He has to go with a carer. They just did a production and they couldn't get him on the stage, he had to sit at the front, so even though they try really hard to get him integrated he is still on the outside a bit.' In other situations, simply attending social venues is problematic. Sharon describes how difficult it is for Zoë to go to the local cinema, 'If I want to take her to the cinema, the disabled seats are about four feet from the screen, right at the front. Then they've got stairs all the way up the middle. So I have to take her out of her chair and walk her up the stairs because she can't sit in the front because it's too big and too loud. Having to sit right at the front you miss half of what goes on and you re straining you're neck because it's too close. There's 12 screens and it's the same in every one.'

In other cases there are organisational barriers to children accessing opportunities. For example, Zak was unable to attend a weekend school trip to an outdoor activities centre because his overnight assisted ventilation could not be facilitated, although he would have been able to participate in all the activities during the day. Cheryl was able to arrange to be with him overnight to supervise his ventilation, but because the parents' room in the complex where the children were staying was already booked, there was nowhere for her to stay with him and he could not sleep in the dormitory with his ventilator and Cheryl supervising him. The school were also unsure about Cheryl staying because it was felt that 'the other children's parents aren't going to be there so they'll be upset when they see Zak's Mum'. Cheryl offered to stay with Zak in a hotel nearby so that he could join in the daytime activities, but this was not permitted, so Zak was unable to participate.

There may also be problems with children being afforded social opportunities because professionals or those organising support services do not understand their importance. Alison recalls explaining to a consultant that when she takes Peter out in the car she needs a second adult with her in case he sleeps: 'He said to me that I'd have to keep him at home. I was like "Yeah, right." Even a child with serious problems, who can't do anything at all, can go out, and you're telling me a little boy who can do all the usual things a toddler does can't go out?'

Peer Relationships

Children who have complex and continuing health needs should have opportunities to develop relationships with their peers, not only for their own good, but for their peers benefit as well. For instance, Evelyn describes how 'Siobhan loves school, she is so popular it would bring a tear to your eye. All her friends just come running to her.' The college which Christian attends also highlight in his reports not only his achievements and his determination, but the contribution which he makes to his peers' lives: 'There is no student at this college who works harder than this popular young man...Christian's development of verbal skills has facilitated his need to initiate communication with a wider circle of communication partners. His sensitive awareness of other students' situations and needs together with this evolving ability to make verbal contact with them, has resulted in Christian's peers being encouraged to achieve even more, and has generally enhanced the enjoyment and motivation of the session for everyone concerned.' Even where the child's contribution is not so obvious, it is important to see that they give a great deal. Despite being immobile, and his communication being very restricted, Jo comments that Mitchell has had a profound effect on many people and he exudes an inner strength and calm which affects others.

Children with complex and continuing health needs may, nonetheless, encounter barriers to forming peer relationships. This may be because their specific needs make communication difficult, or because of their changed opportunities for social interactions. Sometimes it may also be because their condition affects their level of awareness and ability to interact with their peers. As Judy explains, 'it is difficult for Simon to form friendships because of the nature of his disability'. However, since starting a ketogenic diet, Simon's level of awareness has improved. Judy describes how 'if he is next to someone at school you can almost see them talking to each other, he is more aware'. It took Judy some time to persuade medical staff to allow Simon to try a ketogenic diet, and this improvement, as well as the improvement in his epilepsy, illustrates the importance of considering the whole child when making decisions.

Children's opportunities to form peer relationships may also be limited because of the treatment they require and the practicalities associated with this. For example, having friends to stay or visiting friends may be difficult for them. Helen explains how 'David goes to the hospice for respite. Not very often, but he has a friend whom he's at school with and they go at the same time. That's the only way they can be together, because his friend couldn't come and stay the night here, and David couldn't go and stay the night there. The staff are brilliant and take them out to the cinema and they have taken them to a football match.'

In other situations, a child having a correct diagnosis and appropriate support or input can be crucial to their ability to form peer relationships. For Michael, once a diagnosis of autistic spectrum disorder was made, he could receive one to one support for one afternoon a week and could attend a nursery where a specific programme was developed for him. Debby describes how 'Michael loved going to nursery, he had an extremely enjoyable time there, and by the time he left his interaction with other children was developing to the point where he knew and recognised several of the others, and would go and try to join their chasing games' (Barrett 2007).

Children's ability to develop peer relationships can also be affected by how education is organised. Sharon explains that going to a special school has meant that 'Zoë doesn't have friends to tea, because she goes to school on transport, and she comes home on transport. The other children don't necessarily live in the area because special schools have a wide catchment area. They have friends at school, but they don't have a circle of friends out of school, so they don't have that after school teatime and play thing.' Although this can be a significant problem, in some cases, families and schools have worked together to try to improve a child's opportunities to be with their peers. Helen recalls how David's school overcame this problem. The school had residential pupils as well as day pupils, and organised social events for the residential pupils that were not usually open to day pupils. However, the school agreed to make an exception so that David could join the residential pupils' activities four evenings a week, and occasionally join them for breakfast. In the final year of school, the residential pupils spend some time in an independent unit, and David was also able to participate in this, which he describes as 'excellent'. Helen explains how this flexibility by the school 'was really good because that gave him a social life that we couldn't find elsewhere'.

Other people's attitudes can also influence a child's ability to engage in and learn about peer relationships. Debby explains that although her own children unquestioningly incorporate Michael into their activities 'one of James' friends excludes Michael when he comes over'. This type of behaviour can mean that children have fewer opportunities to form peer relationships and to learn about their dynamics than other children. For children like Michael, who have had to make additional efforts to engage with their peers, other children excluding them may also discourage or confuse their efforts and learning.

Developing Independence

Children with complex and continuing health needs face a number of barriers to developing independence. In some instances, the degree of physical independence which children can achieve is very limited. For example, Cheryl and Steve are aware that Hannah will always need them to provide for almost every aspect of her physical needs. In other situations children have varying degrees of physical independence, but their condition makes it more problematic for them to learn, as other children might, to be independent of their parents. As Sharon describes: 'Birthday parties: you can't take Zoë there and come away, you have to stay with her, so you never actually get a break and she never gets her independence because you always need to be around.' This may also mean that how a child's maximum independence may be achieved while maintaining the support that they need is a consideration that is not needed for other children. Sharon explains, 'it's a case of thinking, well, do we need to move when she gets to about 14–15 plus, and find something where we could perhaps build a granny annexe so that she's got her independence, and we've got our independence'.

There may also be more problematic issues over whether children and young people are enabled to develop independence through making choices and directing their lives. As Rosemary explains, it is imperative that those who are supporting children are aware that they should be enabled to give as much direction as possible to their own lives. Although they may be physically unable to carry out activities unaided, they should be given the opportunity and encouraged to learn to choose how, by whom, when, and in what activities they wish to engage and receive assistance. Rosemary describes how rare it is for the staff who provide Hollie's support to allow her such opportunities: 'Hollie is not being allowed to direct her own life. To direct what she wants to do each day.' This may be a reflection of the problem of communication being equated with cognitive and decision-making skills: if Hollie cannot speak to make her preferences known, it is assumed that she has no preferences, and no choices are offered to her. This situation is likely to be compounded by a lack of opportunity to make decisions, resulting in individuals becoming less able or inclined to do so.

The number of situations in which parents have had, for many years and at a higher level than other parents, to ensure their child's safety can make letting them go and take their own risks even harder. Helen describes the difficulty of balancing concern for David's well-being and safety with being able to let him take his own risks: 'As our consultant locally said to us, in a year or two's time David's going to be going out on his own, and he won't be saying: "By the way I've got his medical condition." So no one's going to know.' She explains, and David agrees, 'We have been getting better at letting go over the last year or two.'

Summary

Children and young people with complex and continuing health needs should be seen, first and foremost, as children and young people rather than the focus being their medical or technical needs. However, children who have complex and continuing health needs may have difficulty in enjoying the same opportunities and experiences as other children. This can include their opportunities to communicate, engage in play and leisure activities, learn, and have the chance to engage in social activities and develop relationships with their peers. There are often also significant barriers to children and young people achieving independence. Contributory factors to the challenges which children and young people face may be the physical difficulties that they have, the extent to which others appreciate their rights and abilities, and the effort which others are prepared to make to enable them to enjoy these rights. A priority for those supporting children and young people with complex and continuing health needs should be seeking – with them – to overcome barriers to them enjoying the opportunities that they wish to.

Chapter 3

Being the Parent of a Child who has Complex Needs

Being the parent of a child who has complex and continuing health needs can be very different from being the mother or father of another child. Jo recalls how, as Mitchell's mother, 'although as a woman I was being called a mother, and a very committed Mum, I felt I was in a unique situation.'

The aim of this chapter is to provide some insight into the lives and experiences of parents whose children have complex and continuing health needs. Every child and every parent is different, and the intention is not to imply that all the experiences or views described here apply to all parents, but, rather, to highlight experiences and issues that some parents have encountered.

Rewards

Being the parent of a child with complex and continuing health needs is very demanding, but it can also bring significant pleasures and rewards. Many parents describe how enjoying their child and the love which they give and receive should not be lost in concerns about their 'complex needs'. For example, Sharon describes how 'Zoë has the most wonderful smile, and the wickedest sense of humour. Someone once said to me: "Would you like Zoë to be normal?" And I said: "Well, she wouldn't be the person she is." She is a lovely child.' Cheryl and Steve also explain that 'If ever you need a cuddle, Hannah will give you one. She is very very loving.'

Some parents also consider that their child has indirectly enhanced their lives. Val explains that, despite the work associated with being

Catherine's mother, 'there are days when I think Catherine has enriched my life. If I hadn't had Catherine I'd probably have gone back to work more hours and I'd probably be working in the school holidays. I sometimes do think I'm blessed and I sometimes think she has given me much more in my life. Maybe I can think like that because I was 40 when I had her so I'd done my travel and I'd been a Head of Department which was my aim for work, so I am happy to take a lesser role now and I appreciate all the good things in life more.' Parents also describe how their child has given them the opportunity to meet people whom they would not otherwise have met. For example, Steve and Cheryl explain, 'we have met wonderful people through online communities, namely Special Kids in the UK'.

Parents also describe being enabled to develop or become more aware of personal qualities. For instance, Evelyn is conscious of becoming 'a more patient person, and more involved with my children than I was with my first daughter'. Val has found that because of having to meet Catherine's needs she has learnt a lot about herself, and found that they are quite resourceful. Some parents also describe becoming more broad-minded. Evelyn explains that she has 'learned to never judge people. If a child is having a tantrum, I don't make a judgement, because you don't know what is going on. A lot of children have hidden disabilities. You don't know what is happening, so you can't judge.' Chris also describes how 'there is a lot of prejudice, and also people who just don't think. I was probably like that before. If you haven't had that experience, you don't always think.'

Bringing Your Child Home

In many cases, children with complex and continuing health needs spend a considerable period of time in hospital early in their lives: Siobhan spent her first 81 days of life in hospital; Mollie was five months old when she came home; Michael came home when he was 22 weeks and 5 days; David spent his first 17 months in hospital; and Peter was in hospital for the first nine months of his life. Zak was admitted to hospital when he was three weeks old and did not return home until he was 14 months, his sister Sophia was admitted at ten days of age and came home again when she was six months old.

When a baby is in hospital for a prolonged period of time, their parents' initial experience of being a mother or father, and their early relationship with their child, is very different from that of parents whose babies are at home. This is discussed in more detail in Chapter 4, in relation to premature babies; however, the extent to which parents can participate in their baby's care, the amount and quality of time which they can spend with them, and the degree to which they are included in their baby's life and enabled to feel ownership of their baby may be altered. These points are illustrated by Debby's remark on taking Michael home: 'At long last I was going to get to be a Mum to my son' (Barrett 2007).

The experience of early parenting when a baby is in hospital may include parents having one child in hospital and others at home, necessitating compromises on the time which they can spend with each of their children. For example, David had to spend some weeks in a hospital in London, over a hundred miles from his home. Helen and John's other son was two and a half at the time, and Helen describes how 'we would go to London for a couple of days a week'. Sophia needed to be cared for in Stoke on Trent for six months when Zak was three and a half years old. Cheryl recalls, 'My Mum said: "Right you've got two now, you've got to cut yourself in half." So I used to go on a Friday down to Stoke, come back on a Monday morning, be at home Monday and Tuesday with Zak, take him with me on Wednesday morning on the train, because I didn't want him to miss out on seeing his sister, take him for the day bring him back at teatime, stay at home Thursday and go back on Friday. I had to take him on the train with all his equipment.'

Before their baby can come home, parents often have to contend with a level of planning and practical preparations which other parents do not have to consider. As well as waiting until their baby's medical condition is sufficiently stable for them to come home, parents have to learn how to use equipment and perform health-related tasks for their child. They also often have to adapt their homes or relocate. For example, Cheryl had to move to a house that had space for the equipment which Zak needed and which had easy access to the children's hospital in case of an emergency. Although relocation is not always necessary, finding space for equipment and supplies in their homes is a common problem for parents, as is managing the numerous other practical implications of their child's needs. For instance, Debby describes having to organise obtaining prescriptions from the GP; finding a chemist who supplied oxygen cylinders; organising household and car insurance that would accommodate Michael's needs; informing the fire brigade, the gas and electricity companies before he could come home.

Awaiting the organisation of support services and training of the staff who are needed to support families can also delay a child coming home from hospital. Helen recalls that finding and training staff was one of the main reasons for the delay in David's discharge from hospital: 'It was a case of they had never had a child like this in this area, and had never had to set up this kind of thing and we kept being told we had to be patient.' In addition to finding staff to provide support, funding the support can be problematic, as Helen explains: 'We were told that home care would be expensive. Although inpatient care is more expensive, the money comes from a different pot.' Similarly, Alison explains that, because of 'the lack of forward thinking and long-term planning', Peter remained in hospital long after Alison was confident about providing his care while funding for the support he would need at home was agreed. For parents this means that their baby being able to come home appears to be a matter of economic expediency and organisational politics.

Because of the complexity of the care which some children need, and the length of time that they have spent in hospital, despite the pleasure of them coming home, it can be daunting for their parents. Debby describes how although 'it was wonderful to have Michael home, walking out of the hospital was an amazing feeling'. At the same time, 'coming home with Michael was a mixture of fantastic and terrifying' (Barrett 2007). Tracy also recalls that bringing Mollie home was 'fantastic. Scary, but fantastic.'

Expertise

Parents all describe having to become knowledgeable about their child's condition, and becoming accustomed to a range of medical and technical aspects of their care. Because they carry out their child's care every day, make decisions about their needs and responses to treatment and care, they become experts in this and their knowledge and expertise often exceeds that of many professionals. Debby explains: 'We are the ones who have known Michael from day one. We are the only ones who go with him to all his appointments, to every doctor, we are the only ones who juggle and watch things every day.' Alison describes how, because of its rarity, many staff do not fully understand the implications of Peter's condition in the way that she does: 'When he has been very very poorly and they say: "No, he's fine," it's getting them to try to understand what his condition means. Like if he has cold, or when he had RSV [respiratory synctial virus], they said: "Oh but his respiratory rate is still the same," and you're like "because he's got congenital central hypoventilation syndrome, so his respiratory rate won't respond to any extra stress." It's things like that. You have to look at things differently.'

The expert knowledge and skills that parents develop, and the health-related roles which they take on can, nonetheless, detract from their expected role as a parent. One aspect of this can be them having to perform unpleasant procedures for their child, which contrasts with the expected nurturing and protecting role of a parent. Chris recalls that he and Tracy used to have to 'suction Mollie's nose, which she hated, but at the end of the day, you had to do it, to make her better'. Such responsibilities can also mean that parents feel that the time they spend in their parenting role is diluted by their healthcare role. Evelyn describes how 'it would be nice sometimes just to be Siobhan's Mum. After I had Siobhan, I had my little boy and I always felt like I had forgotten to do something because he didn't need anything doing: changing nappies and things, but no therapies; for Siobhan there was always treatment or therapy from the day she came home from hospital. It would be nice sometimes to just be her mum.'

The expert knowledge of their child's medical and technical needs that parents develop can also affect how others perceive them. Debby notes that learning to speak 'the language' of complex care has been essential but 'in some cases learning the language doesn't do you any favours. I've been accused of being very clinical about Michael, because I use clinical terms, terms I've had to learn over the years for the conditions he's got because those are the names for them. But then I am accused of being clinical.' On the other hand, without this knowledge Debby's communication with health and social care professionals and systems would be even harder than it is now.

Parents' understanding of their child's condition and the implications of this can also be an emotional burden which they have to carry. Jo explains that she is fully aware of the frailty of Mitchell's life: 'I call it "Going to the edge": I've been to the edge, and I know, I don't know, but I do have a sense of what it will be like when the moment happens. I've been that close, and it's a horrible place. It's knowledge that I wish I didn't have. We have literally peered over the edge, and I just don't know what's going to happen when it actually happens. When we fall off. It's a dreadful feeling: horrible.'

As well as knowledge of specific aspects of their child's care, parents universally describe knowing their child or children much better than anyone else does. Cheryl explains, 'nobody knows the child better than the parent, especially a child with special needs'. This includes intuitive knowledge of their child's cues, responses, and state of being, and awareness of very small, subtle signs from their child. For instance, Alison describes how she has a feeling with Peter, so if she says something, they should listen because she's right. 'With him if something is wrong I just have a feeling. And every time I have had that feeling I've been right. It's like a jigsaw and one piece is missing. Something's not quite right.'

Practicalities

The needs which many children have mean that their parents have to be extremely well organised and often have very little flexibility in their days. As Jo explains: 'Your daytime has to be very regimented because Mitchell needs things doing at certain times.' Alongside organising all the day-to-day care that their children need, parents have to juggle attending appointments related to their needs, which can span a range of specialities and locations. In some cases children have to attend specialist centres which involves travel and time away from home. Given the difficulties that taking some children out occasion, and especially when there is more than one child in the family, this can create major logistical problems. For example, Rachel describes how, when Emmy had an appointment at a specialist children's hospital in London, the whole family went to London, which meant taking the other three girls out of school and finding overnight accommodation.

Alongside meeting the child's routine day-to-day needs, their parents have to be constantly vigilant: aware of the risks which their child's condition carries, and of all possible eventualities, in all situations, and build in time and strategies to manage these. As Jo explains, 'you have to be mindful of things at all times'. Some children require constant supervision because of their inability to maintain their own safety, which restricts what their parents can do 24 hours a day, even during periods when the child requires no specific input. For example, because of his tracheostomy Mitchell cannot be left without direct supervision, so when Jo is alone with him she, 'can't go upstairs because he can't be left for longer than a couple of minutes'. Chris and Tracy also recall what it was like when Mollie first came home: 'We couldn't leave her for a minute, even if we were going to the toilet. She was on so much oxygen that if she pulled it off she would go blue.' Lucy needs two adults to be available at all times. If for any reason this is not possible she has to be in bed, because this is the only way that her care and risks can be managed by one person. Other children do not require constant direct supervision, but do require a higher level of supervision or a greater degree of assistance to participate in activities than another child of their age. For example, Sharon explains: 'If Zoë says "Mummy I want to come and help you wash up" you have to think of the logistics: I've got to get a chair out there, make sure there's plastic stuff in the sink, stand behind her and help her, and as much as you think it's lovely for her to do it, it takes about four times as long. You're permanently giving things the level of thought you give to organising things for a much younger child.'

Other children may not appear to require close supervision, but their parents have to be aware of the risks that their condition carries and constantly plan for these to ensure that they are safe. Helen describes what happened when David went on a camping trip: 'I went over to do the nights and took all the equipment and I was talking to the person who organised it. She was saying that out of all the children (who are all from a school for children with physical disabilities or medical needs), if you watched them, you would say David is the most able and why is he here. But when we risk-assessed them, David was at the greatest risk because it is life-threatening. If he did the assault course and knocked himself unconscious, he would stop breathing. He is the one who helps out with everything, and helps the other pupils, but, on risk assessment, he is at the greatest risk.'

The level of many children's needs means that these have to be taken into account in every part of their parents' lives, and what another parent might do almost unthinkingly can take considerable time and effort. For example, Jo explains, 'you can't nip to the shops. Like yesterday, I wanted some milk, but if you're going to the shop you've got to let the ramp down, pack all the things, get Mitchell into the car, drive there, take him out of the car, go in the shop, put him back in the car again, come back and its all so much of a faff.'

Even when children are not with their parents, for example when they are at school, because of their expert knowledge and a lack of other back-up services their parents are often contacted with queries, and need to be available to take over their child's care if a problem arises. This means that they are effectively 'on call' for 24 hours a day, seven days a week, 365 days a year.

As well as their daytimes having to be very organised, in many cases, parents' sleep is disturbed for much longer than would be the case with another child. Zak, Sophia, David, Peter and Mitchell require constant supervision at night, and unless they have overnight carers, their parents get little or no sleep. Even then, the carers cannot always deal with all eventualities and parents' sleep remains subject to disruption. For example, Zak and Sophia have a carer at night, but if their ventilation requires adjustment 'some carers can't do anything like that, so you're up and down doing that. We have a couple (of carers) who have been here before Sophia was born but with most carers you'll be up and down. If they're slightly unwell you have them (the carer) knocking at your bedroom door.' In other cases, even though their child does not require constant supervision, their needs can interrupt their parents' sleep. For instance, Emmy requires overnight apnoea monitoring and the alarm sounds frequently, often for false alarms, but as Rachel explains she, 'can't take that risk of not going in'.

This combination of planning for and meeting their child's needs means that parents often have very little time for themselves. Mr and Mrs Hethrington describe having no time even for simple luxuries, such as a soak in a bath, or to do their shopping at leisure. Jo describes how easy it would be to 'drown' in simply getting everything done. She suggests that 'in order to get close to living the life that I would want for myself as a person, there's a hell of a lot to do first, so I have to be extremely organised, extremely committed to being organised and getting everything done, and once I've done that I can do the me bit. But there is a hell of a lot to do to get to that point, and in order to do that I have to be very determined.'

Because of the impact on every aspect of their lives, 24 hours a day, the situation in which parents are placed is very different from the workload for the staff who provide care for their children. As Val explains, being a part of the team that provides Catherine's respite care, in a unit designed for this purpose, is very different from caring for Catherine at home because the staff do not have the usual running of a household, looking after another child, working, shopping, and so on to do at the same time. In addition, their shifts last for 8–12 hours, not 24, and ensuring that the respite centre has everything needed to look after Catherine is Val's responsibility as they do not keep supplies of anything.

Administration

As well as the physical practicalities and organisational issues concerning their child's direct care, parents often spend a considerable amount of time in administration related to their child. Cheryl describes how 'you do become a sort of secretary. It's a whole new role. It's not just being a Mum, it's being a Mum, a secretary and a Filofax.' Rosemary explains that this aspect of her role includes liaison between services, discussions about staffing, and seeking services, equipment and specialists who can assist with Hollie's and Christian's needs, as well as attending appointments and meetings. Because some of Mitchell's funding is provided by direct payments, Jo's workload includes managing the payments and a staff rota, 'and if someone can't come you have to find someone else at short notice'.

Cheryl describes how, because the administrative element of her role includes having to manage Hannah's money for her, this adds an emotional element to her work: she feels guilty at spending her child's money. She explains how 'for birthday and Christmas she always gets money, and recently I have got quite a few things for her, like a comfy chair from the special needs catalogue. But I feel so guilty going in and taking money out of her account. I feel I have to justify why I'm taking it out. We haven't got the money to buy all the special things for her so if she's got the money sitting there, and its going to make her life better, make her more comfortable, we use it, but I do feel guilty.'

Another part of many parents' role is obtaining and organising supplies. For example, Catherine's family has half a garage full of her supplies, and Val has to spend some time every day in ordering, keeping track of stocks, checking deliveries, being in for deliveries, and making sure that established stocks continue to match Catherine's needs. Most of the supplies are collected or delivered in monthly batches, with the exception of the sterile water which is required for Catherine's gastro-jejunostomy tube. This is provided weekly. Val explains: 'We get a month's worth of milk, nappies; everything else is delivered in reasonable amounts and I have worked it out over the years so that everything arrives in a reasonable timeframe, as closely as possible together. The GP and I have tried to work it out between us so that we pretty much do a prescription a month. But we can only have a week's supply of sterile water at a time.' The impracticality of this variation is clear, and incorporating weekly stock checks and deliveries adds to Val's already overwhelming workload.

The amount of administration and organisation involved in being the parent of a child with complex and continuing health needs means that it is often hard for parents to switch off. Rosemary describes the most distressing area of being Hollie and Christian's mother as being at night: 'When you're trying to get to sleep, it is all the flashbacks of the things that have gone wrong during the day. What happened, what you said, what you should have said to have put your point over more effectively, and what you're going to say, and who you're going to write to. The flashbacks are so vivid and so real that by the morning you don't know if you really said that or sent the email or not. Often, I can actually visualise myself writing letters. In the morning you think: "Was that real?"'

Going out

Taking out children who have complex and continuing health needs can present a challenge for their parents. Debby describes going out with Michael as 'like going out on manoeuvres'. The level of planning which can be needed is illustrated by the equipment, medication and supplies which Catherine requires if she goes out for a day. This includes: syringes for aspirating Catherine's gastrojejunostomy tube; syringes for winding her; syringes for any drugs that she needs and to flush the tube; the pump through which her feeds and water are given; her medications; her feeds; sterile water; nappies; wipes, and so on. Despite parents achieving a high level of organisation, things can still go wrong, with more dramatic effect than would be the case for many children. Debby recalls: 'I have run out of oxygen while I am out and then you're searching in a panic for a chemist who can swap the oxygen over because the supposedly full oxygen cylinder was, in fact, empty.' As with the day-to-day organisation of events, taking out children includes thinking about things that may not be needed, but which parents must, nonetheless, have available. Helen recalls: 'Last week, we knew we were going a long way in the car and I said we really should put a ventilator in the back of the car in case he has a sleep.'

Taking out a child can also be physically demanding. If children have mobility problems, as they get older, their weight and the equipment that they require can make taking them out more difficult. Jo explains: 'I find it physically harder now. Not just lifting, but changing and moving position. When we go out, we have to go to places that don't involve going up hills. We are real out-and-about people. We love being out and about, and Mitchell loves being out and about, going to the park and stuff, and now I find it really hard to go to the park on my own because he is heavy to push.'

Long-term Responsibility

When a child has complex and continuing health needs it often means that their parents have to provide for them for longer, and at a very different level, than other parents. Jo describes how, with other children, when a stage is exhausting 'you know that you're going to move from, for example, the getting up in the night. There's light at the end of the tunnel. But for a child, who isn't developing in that way, it lasts a hell of a long time.' Cheryl also explains: 'It's a harsh realisation because every now and then I think: "This is it, for ever, its never going to go away." Hannah will always need us. It is nice, in one way, in that she'll always be my little girl, but there is a difference. On the other hand, I will always know where she is, I won't have to worry what she is up to or where she is when she's 18. But I won't get my identity back in the same way as other Mums.'

Having a child with complex and continuing health needs also means that their parents always need to be well enough and have the energy to facilitate their needs. Val explains: 'What worries me hugely is what would happen if I were ever to become ill. Because even the most qualified nurse couldn't just step in without knowing Catherine's routine.' Mrs Hethrington has recently been diagnosed as having a painful skin condition. Even when her hands are too sore to wash up, she has to get Lucy up, bath her, change her, dress her, and draw up and administer drugs and feeds. As she explains, if she were in paid employment, she would have been off sick for the past five months, but she continues her 'work' caring for Lucy because there is no alternative.

Emotional Demands

As well as the physical and organisational demands of caring for a child with complex and continuing health needs, there is a significant emotional element to being their parent. As Debby states, for many parents, 'this journey is a very rocky road to take, there are no easy answers and no easy solutions, it leaves you physically and mentally exhausted'.

The emotional element of having a child with complex needs may relate to past events, as Chris explains with Mollie approaching her second birthday: 'Even now, you get times when your eyes well up for no reason, when you look back and think.' Parents may also have to live with their knowledge of the frailty of their child's life. Jo describes this as 'living in sort of suspense. I am definitely aware of...not waiting for it to happen, but being aware that it's going to happen.' This means that, despite the effort needed to care for Mitchell, Jo would have it no other way: 'I recognise that this is the best bit. Because when eventually something does happen to him, it will never be the same, and I will always be looking back, to when he was here, because it will change for ever in a way that I don't want it to change. I'd rather juggle everything, however hard it is, because if I didn't have to juggle everything Mitchell would have to have died, and I don't want that. But that's on the horizon for me all the time. It's there.' Some parents also describe feeling guilt or responsibility for their child's needs. For example, Rachel explains: 'I do feel it's [Emmy's needs] my fault, I shouldn't have had another child. They said there was no reason [for her babies being born prematurely], but I do feel it is my fault.'

Another emotional element of having a child with complex and continuing health needs can be dealing with losses. Debby explains how ongoing losses and grieving have become a part of her life: 'You grieve for what you expected with a newborn baby, the whole neonatal experience, for what might have been, what could have happened. Then, it's OK, because you think he will get better, and you set up plans for the magic age of two, and then you grieve for the child you were going to get at two as well. Then you think, well, maybe because he was so premature, and so ill, and he was hardly home the first year, so maybe it will take until three.'

However, as Debby recalls, when Michael was finally diagnosed as having autistic spectrum disorder, another wave of grief swept in as the family 'kissed ever having "normal" goodbye that day, and once again I'm left grieving for the baby/child I never had' (Barrett 2007). Jo also describes how losses can accumulate over time. She felt no loss at Mitchell's initial disability, but has experienced two major losses since in her life with Mitchell. The first was when Mitchell had a gastrostomy performed, which meant that he could no longer be a part of family mealtimes, Jo could no longer the cook meals that he liked, and it removed one of the pleasures in Mitchell's life. The second loss related to Mitchell having his tracheostomy, after which he could no longer be left alone, even for a few minutes. The family thus had to have the necessary but intrusive presence of staff in their home, additional equipment was required wherever they went, holidays became almost impossible, and there were suddenly some things that Mitchell could no longer be involved in because he had a tracheostomy.

In many cases, expected aspects of parenting are lost and parents have to make adjustments to their existing lives in ways that may seem small, but, nonetheless constitute a loss. Hannah used a wheelchair at the age of two, and Cheryl recalls, 'it got to the point where she was uncomfortable we were like, right, it's time to use the wheelchair now. It does take time to adjust to the idea of: "Why can't she sit in this lovely Mamas and Papas thing that we bought that cost £400?" But she can't.' Cheryl and Steve also explain how, despite the pleasure that Hannah gives them, her needs have meant them making changes in their possessions and lifestyle. For example, 'it's the little things you don't think about: we had to get rid of our gorgeous Golf GT–TDI that we had from brand new. Now I have a people carrier. It's not that I resent it, but it is a change in your life that you didn't expect.'

Changes in Role and Identity

Parents may feel that their identity changes significantly when they become the mother or father of a child with complex and continuing health needs. This may include changes in the way in which they have to behave to ensure that their child's needs are met. Sharon explains: 'It's always a case of what you want you have to fight for. It's whoever shouts loudest gets.' Val also describes how she has 'become more assertive because Catherine's got no one else to speak up for her, to fight her corner'. However, this is often at odds with the way in which people have previously had to behave, and their perceptions of themselves. As Judy explains, 'I am not naturally a pushy parent. But that is how you have to be.'

Parents' social interactions and opportunities may also be altered. Debby describes how 'you go from having a life that is fairly well organised, and you have time to have a life, to suddenly finding yourself in this world full of medical people and equipment and everything else just goes'. Cheryl explains that for the past ten years she has been unable to go out in the evening: 'The carers don't start until half past nine, so if the other Mums at school say they're going out at seven o'clock, I can't, and by the time I'd be ready to come out everyone's coming home.' Activities which were important to parents often cease to be possible: Mr Hethrington recounts how, because of Lucy's needs, 'my life stopped'. His passion was motorbikes. He used to go out on his bike, and teach his son about bikes every Saturday and Sunday. But 'it got to stage when I couldn't go out with Ryan'. Now for leisure activities the most he can do is go to the club on corner of the road for a few hours on days when Lucy has respite care. This lack of time or opportunity to do a great deal more than care for their child means that families often find it difficult to keep in contact with friends or relatives. Debby explains, 'we have become very insular because our lives revolve around Michael and his needs' (Barrett 2007).

In addition to lack of time being a problem, parents may not have opportunities to meet other parents. When children attend special school this alters the interactions which parents have with one other. As Sharon describes: 'You're not at the school gate talking, because the children are all on transport. So sometimes you can feel very very isolated, because you don't know anybody else.' Families may also become isolated because they no longer share common ground with previous friends and acquaintances, or because friends cannot manage the differences in their lives. Sharon explains how 'quite a few became our ex-friends now, I suppose, when Zoë became noticeably different; although they were the same age, because Zoë couldn't do the same things as their children, they suddenly dropped out. So we've got no contact with them now. Fine, their loss, but then you suddenly don't have a circle of friends.' Debby also describes how Michael's needs means that much of the common ground which she has with her peers has been lost, not only in relation to their children, but because of their outlook on life and priorities: 'I find it difficult to mix with others, because the things that others worry about sometimes seem so trivial to me, part of it is also not being able to deal with other people's worries and concerns' (Barrett 2007).

Being the mother or father of a child with complex and continuing health needs can be so all-consuming that the parents' own identity becomes subsumed in this role. Cheryl explains: 'You do lose your identity a bit. I have just come to realise that in the past few months. We were talking about plastic surgery, and I said I'm going to have everything put back where it should be: my boobs put back and my stomach put back and everyone said: "Why?" and I said to my friend, who also has a little boy, "When he's 18 or 25 or at some point, he's going to leave home, and you will go back to being you, you can go out on a night out and get as drunk as you like or do whatever you like: you can just be you, and do whatever you want." But I'm never ever ever going to be me again, because Hannah's going to be needing me and Steve for as long as we can care for her. I'm a firm believer in the fact that she's our daughter and we care for her, but I am never going to get me back, I am always going to be Hannah's Mum. Even when she's 40, I'm going to be Hannah's Mum. It wouldn't be like that ordinarily. So for me, if I can get myself back to feeling like me, I am going to have my boobs put back and my tummy taken in if that's what it takes.'

As well as their identity, parents' own needs become secondary to those of their child. While this may be the case with all children, the level of the child's need and the time that caring for a child with complex and continuing health needs takes means that this often has a greater effect for their parents. For example, Rachel explains that juggling her four girls' appointments and needs means that she often misses or cannot arrange her own outpatient appointments related to a cardiac condition. Although this lack of time to meet parents' own needs is often caused by the sheer workload of their children's needs, it may also be that parents' needs are seen as unimportant by service providers. As Alison describes: 'We do a very good job and sometimes you're treated a bit as if you don't matter. The child matters but you're just the parent.'

In addition to changes in their own sense of identity and ability to meet their own needs, other people's perceptions of parents may be changed because of their role in their child's care. Val describes how other people generally see her primarily as Catherine's mother: 'When I go out all I talk about is Catherine, that's often all people want to talk about, so you lose your identity. I want to talk about other things; I do have opinions about other things.'

Employment

Many parents find that their child's needs alter their ability to engage in paid employment. Alison explains: 'You have plans when you have a child, how you're going to go back to work part-time, and then when he's at school increase your hours.' However, when the child has complex and continuing health needs, these plans often change dramatically. Alison has taken a five-year career break. Although she describes herself as fortunate in that her employer has agreed to this, in the interim five years she is unsalaried and there will be no guarantee of what job Alison will be offered or able to do. She explains: 'You can't give that commitment to an employer. You have a child with complex needs, they will always come first. So I couldn't do a 9–5 job. I'd need a very understanding employer. If he's sick or anything I always have to be on hand.'

The unpredictability of children's needs, combined with a lack of out of school childcare for children with complex and continuing health needs makes employment opportunities for their parents very limited. Sharon describes how 'you are very limited as to what you can do because there is no childcare'. In many cases, both parents can only work if their employers are very flexible. Helen recalls: 'I felt I was unemployable, that I was not reliable enough. I knew that if David was ill and had a cold and couldn't go to school I had no one else I could rely on.' However, she applied for a job with a local support group for people with autism, and was 'very upfront and told them about David and his condition and they were fine and employed me and I've been there ever since, and I love it. They are so flexible.' Val works two mornings a week, and considers that she is 'very lucky to have a term-time contract as I do not have anyone to look after Catherine during the school holidays. I would not be able to work otherwise. I am really lucky I work in such a supportive environment.'

In some cases, it is impossible for either of a child's parents to work because of their child's needs. Mr and Mrs Hethrington's employment options are virtually non-existent. During school holidays, they both need to be with Lucy all day. When she is at school they both need to be present until she leaves the house, and to be there when she returns. If Lucy is unwell, or anything prevents a nurse being at the school, Lucy cannot attend, and her parents both need to be at home with her. If Lucy has appointments, one parent has to drive and the other travels with them in case Lucy needs anything. This leaves relatively little time when either of them can work.

Changes in employment status can have a significant effect on parents' self-perception and well-being. Mr Hethrington explains that he had to give up the job which he loved because, with Lucy's increasing incapacity, he was too far away from home too often, but he would like to work. He describes how a period of time during which he was able to get short-term work did him an amazing amount of good mentally. Helen also describes how important being able to go back to work was for her, and how, after returning to work she was a completely different person: 'That was just what I needed. I couldn't have stayed at home, I just felt really boring.' Judy was unable to pursue a career until 18 months ago: 'I got to the point that all I had done was stay at home and look after Simon, and although I love him, I needed to do something for myself.' Val describes how her hours at work are the one time when she can be someone other than Catherine's mother: 'When I'm there, those eight hours that I'm at work, I'm not Catherine's Mum. I feel respected at work.' In addition, work can provide a welcome relief from the constant demands and isolation of caring for a child with complex and continuing health needs. Val explains, 'also, we have a laugh at work and I don't find much to laugh about at home all day'.

Summary

Having a child with complex and continuing health needs can be very demanding for their parents. As Helen describes: 'Looking back now, if someone had told us "Your son's going to have this rare condition and you're going to have to cope with this," I would have said no, we couldn't cope. And looking back I think: "How did I do that?" But you just do.' The challenges which many parents face include their child being in hospital for a prolonged period, often soon after they are born; the difficulties associated with juggling being involved in the care of one child in hospital and others at home; organising their child's discharge home; the complexity of managing their day-to-day practical needs; the administration and planning involved in their care; the long-term and unrelenting nature of their child's needs, and the long-term responsibility that this carries; and the emotional demands of having a child with complex and continuing health needs. Parents often experience significant changes in their own lives because of their child's needs, including alterations in their employment status and career structure, changes to their self-identity and the way in which other perceive them. However, despite the often unrelenting nature of caring for their child, many parents also describe the rewards and benefits which their child has brought to their lives.

As well as rising to these challenges and accommodating significant changes to their lives, parents often have to develop knowledge and expertise in medical and technical procedures. Their knowledge of their child's condition and needs, as well as their finely tuned and intuitive knowledge of the child, means that they can usually provide professionals with a highly reliable indication of the child's condition, which should not be dismissed. As Alison explains: 'You do come to a stage where you do become more knowledgeable about your child's condition than anyone, and they shouldn't take that away from you.'

Chapter 4

Premature Babies

Some children who develop complex and continuing health needs are born prematurely and require intensive care during the neo-natal period. The effects of prematurity are only some of the reasons for children developing long-term health problems; neither do all premature babies develop long term health problems. However, the increasing number of babies who survive extremely premature birth means that the concerns which this raises for children and their families are very relevant.

This chapter explores the experiences of four parents whose babies were born prematurely: Michael was born at 24 weeks' gestation; Siobhan was born at 28 weeks; Jodie was born at 30 weeks; Bethany at 26 weeks; and Niahm and Emmy at 25 weeks. Bailey and Mollie were born at 26 weeks.

Meeting Your Critically Ill Newborn Baby

When a baby is born extremely prematurely, their parents' immediate meeting and bonding with them is different from their expectations. Parents are sometimes unable to see or hold their baby immediately after they are born. Rachel remembers 'putting my arms out to hold Jodie and I was told I couldn't' as Jodie would be going to the neo-natal intensive care nursery (Dickinson 2007). Debby and Martin did not see Michael for almost three hours after he was born, Rachel was not able to see Emmy until the day after she was born, and Evelyn was unable to see Siobhan until the day after her birth because she was herself unwell.

When parents do see their baby, their size and vulnerability are often overwhelming. Evelyn describes how 'I took one look at her and just broke down. I remember thinking "how can something so small and fragile possibly survive?"' (Young and Young 2007). Debby also recounts how Michael 'looked like a scrap of nothing, he was so small, perfectly formed but, oh, so small. His eyes were fused shut, he was wearing the biggest nappy I have ever seen, and yet this was a nappy designed for prem babies' (Barrett 2007). When a baby requires intensive care, as well as their appearance, the sight and sounds of the equipment that is needed to sustain them can be overpowering. Debby describes: 'When we did get into there [the neonatal intensive care unit; NICU] the whole room caved in on me, and all I could see was the wires, monitors, alarms, and the ventilator. There were tubes, syringes, lots of high-tech-looking equipment, which made a lot of noise, and somewhere in among all this, under a plastic bag, was my son' (Barrett 2007).

This combination of the baby's size and the bank of equipment, which indicates the severity of the their condition, can give parents a sense of helplessness, personally and for their baby. Rachel describes how 'I have been there, watching a stranger breathe for my child, and knowing I have to trust a person I don't know' (Dickinson 2007). Debby also recalls: 'Seeing your child fighting for it's very existence, knowing that there is nothing you can do to help. Your child is totally dependent on the machines and the nurses and doctors' (Barrett 2007).

This combination of sights, sounds, feelings and being aware of their baby's vulnerability means that the emotions that parents of critically ill newborn babies feel may be very different from what they expect or are expected to feel. Debby describes her feelings when she first saw Michael: 'I didn't feel an overwhelming love and desire for this little scrap. What I felt I can only describe as fear.' Debby recalls her parents coming to visit and the 'look of sheer pride and amazement on both their faces as they looked at this tiny perfect baby'. In contrast, 'all I could see was machines' (Barrett 2007).

Being the Parents of a Premature Baby

Having a baby who is born prematurely and whom requires intensive care changes the expected experience of early parenthood. Rachel's recollection of being on the post-natal ward after Bethany was born illustrates the contrast between her experience and that of other parents: 'I could see mums and dads cuddling their new arrivals in the beds opposite me. It was horrible. I was in a strange place, miles away from my family, and didn't even know how my baby was doing' (Dickinson 2007).

In some cases, parents can barely even touch their newborn baby. Debby recalls that Michael 'did not like being handled or touched by anyone, his oxygen saturations would drop when touched, and the nurses learnt to leave him well alone, which meant that we too were not able to touch him' (Barrett 2007). Debby and Martin had their first cuddle with Michael when he was eight weeks old. Emmy was 15 days old and still receiving assisted ventilation when Rachel held her for the first time. Rachel's description illustrates how, even when parents can touch and hold their baby, this is very different from other parents' experience of holding their newborn baby for the first time: 'To hold you was wonderful but scary at the same time' (Dickinson 2007).

The difficulty in handling extremely premature babies can mean that parents miss being involved in providing the care that they would expect to give their baby, for example changing nappies, bathing and dressing them. Debby explains: 'I couldn't do anything for him, anything he needed the nurses did. I just sat, and stared at the machines. No one thought to ask us if we wanted to do his cares, mouthcare, nappy care, and so on. He was nine weeks old before we were offered that opportunity.'

In many cases, parents have to juggle the time that they have between their newborn baby and other children. This can mean that important childcare opportunities may be missed because activities are carried out when they are, of necessity, not present. For example, Michael's first bath was given by the nurses, while the family were not there. Debby reports that 'they opened the incubator and thought he needed a bath. The smell hit them, so the nurse bathed him.' The family was given a photograph of the event. Although parents may miss out on their child's care because they are away from the hospital when things need to be done, this is not always the reason. It appears that staff do not always appreciate the importance of parents being fully involved in and having ownership of their baby and their care. While Debby and Michael were not there when it was decided that Michael needed his first bath, his second bath was given by a nurse while Debby watched but was told she could not do it. Similarly, with Michael's feeding there appears to have been a lack of appreciation of the importance of parents being enabled to do as much of their baby's care as is possible. Debby recalls that not only was Michael's first feed given by the nurses, but that thereafter she often found that staff on the special care baby unit (SCBU) 'fed Michael when they knew we were coming in' (Barrett 2007).

As well as parents being given the chance to feed their baby, feeding premature babies is often very different from parents' expectations of feeding their baby. In many cases the baby cannot, at least initially, take breast or bottle feeds. For example, none of Rachel's daughters were able to take oral feeds immediately, although they all had expressed breast milk via nasogastric tubes. Emmy was 55 days old when she had her first attempt at breastfeeding, and establishing feeding was difficult because she found it hard to co-ordinate breathing and feeding, and to tolerate her feeds. She was later found to have gross reflux.

As well as missing out on physical aspects of their care, the baby's survival being uncertain from minute to minute produces an almost unimaginable emotional charge for their parents, at a time when other families are celebrating a newborn baby's birth. This can affect how far parents dare to bond with their newborn baby. As Debby explains, her fear of losing Michael meant that she did not dare to engage fully with him: 'I was so totally convinced that he was going to die, that in order to protect myself I stayed away emotionally' (Barrett 2007). Sadly, this fear is very real, and not all babies do survive. Chris and Tracy's son, Bailey, died on the neo-natal unit at the age of two weeks.

Parents of critically ill premature babies may not receive the input from friends and family, and the celebration of their baby's birth, which they otherwise would. Debby explains: 'When you have your baby so early, people don't know how to react or respond: do they send cards or don't they?' Parents may also have to contend with thoughtless and hurtful comments about their baby. For example, one of Debby's colleagues described Michael as 'a miscarriage that survived'.

Although having a critically ill premature baby means that parents do not experience a number of expected aspects of early parenting, their experiences are often much more intense than those of other parents. As well as constantly fearing for their baby's life, instead of being able to nurture and protect their baby they have to see them suffer invasive procedures and distress in a way which other parents do not. Debby recalls seeing Michael's ventilator tube being changed: 'As the tube was removed he was terrified...that vision of him still haunts me even now almost seven years later' (Barrett 2007). Being on a neo-natal intensive care unit (NICU) can also be intense and exhausting, the array of equipment, the constant fear for their child's life, and the confined space creating an environment which Tracy and Chris, despite their admiration for the NICU where Bailey and Mollie were cared for, describe as 'so alien'. This is augmented by parents often feeling unable to leave their babies and thus remaining on the unit for 24 hours a day. Chris recalls: 'We actually got told by the staff to go home. We were there for two weeks, without leaving the hospital. We were there 24/7 for two weeks.'

Families can also be isolated from outside support from friends and family, and the support provided by other parents on a NICU is, as Chris describes, 'a lifeline. We used to chat to the other parents. We knew the routine: the doctors round at nine and then all to the coffee room to let off steam, chat, laugh, and cry. That helped a lot. That sounding board and understanding.' Despite this invaluable support, the close environment of the NICU and relationships between families means that the progress of and events associated with other babies can be hugely significant for parents. Debby recalls one baby on the unit who was born at 25 weeks' gestation whom, 'we held as our shining light, our inspiration, if he could do it, then so could Michael'. Debby goes on to explain how, when she and Martin learnt of this baby's death 'we were devastated, not only for him and for his parents, but his death shook our very foundations of security. We will never forget that little boy and the hope and belief that he gave us, in the short time we knew of him' (Barrett 2007).

Although in some cases parents do not feel able to leave the NICU, in others they may be separated from their baby, sometimes by hundreds of miles, because of a lack of NICU cots. This was something which nearly had a devastating effect on Chris and Tracy before their twins were born. Chris explains: 'When Tracy first went in we were told that one [twin] would have to go to Nottingham and one to Norwich, because that unit didn't have the space. We had all that going on even before they are born.' Fortunately, by the time the twins were born, 'it just so happened that two babies were discharged from the unit that day'. So Bailey and Mollie were both cared for in the local NICU.

Where parents have other children, although they want to be with their baby, they often have to divide their time between them and their older children, especially, as is frequently the case, when their baby's stay in hospital is prolonged. Leaving their baby at the NICU can be extremely distressing for parents. Rachel describes how she felt when she had to leave Emmy to be with the rest of her family: 'I hate leaving you behind, especially if you are awake, I can't leave you, I don't like to think I'd deserted you' (Dickinson 2007). In addition, the NICU may be some distance from the family home, making the division of time and parenting even more difficult. Rachel's second daughter, Bethany, was cared for in an NICU about 35 miles from her home. Debby and Martin's home was also approximately 30 miles from the unit where Michael was born.

Facing your Baby's Mortality

When a newborn baby is critically ill, their parents have to consider the possibility that they may not survive. In some cases, where there is the possibility of the baby being born extremely prematurely, this possibility is presented before the baby is born. Debby was advised when she was 20 weeks pregnant that, should they need to deliver her baby before 24 weeks, 'he would be allowed to die' (Barrett 2007). In other instances, the uncertainty over a baby's survival occurs as they are born. When Rachel was 25 weeks pregnant and being monitored Niamh's heart beat became unrecordable. Niamh was delivered by emergency Caesarean section and Rachel describes how, 'I will never forget being put to sleep knowing there was no heartbeat' and then 'being woken to hear that my baby was alive' (Dickinson 2007). The importance of the way in which information about a baby's likely survival is conveyed is not something which professionals should underestimate. Tracy recalls how, when she was 24 weeks pregnant and was admitted to hospital: 'This neo-natal doctor came to see us and said, so matter of factly, "If you have them now, we're not going to do anything." It was so matter of fact. She didn't even say it nicely.' Chris comments: 'I just couldn't believe it. I was speechless. She might as well have just got a sledgehammer and hit me.'

There is often ongoing doubt about the survival of extremely premature babies. Rachel describes her early days in the NICU: 'Emmy would be doing OK one minute, the next they were calling for us to come in. I had so many times with the doctors saying she wasn't going to make it.' Debby recalls her overwhelming memory of Michael's early life as being of constant fear, with every moment potentially holding the news that Michael had died. At night, she recalls, 'lying there in the dark, listening to the sound of footsteps going up and down the corridor. Every so often the phone would ring. I lay there waiting for the door to open, for the visit from a midwife to say that the NICU was on the phone. Again that overwhelming sense of fear. I was absolutely terrified. I wasn't sleeping, I didn't see how anything so small and so dependent on all those machines could live. I would lie in my bed on the ward waiting for the knock on the door, I have never known fear like it.'

Equally, despite the seriousness of their babies' conditions, being thrown into the world of prematurity may be so extreme and events so rapid that parents are unable to take in the severity of their baby's illness and the possible outcomes. Chris describes when Mollie and Bailey were born: 'We didn't have time to comprehend it at all. Really, until we lost Bailey we didn't realise what sort of situation we were in. Until then it didn't compute in our brains. We were on autopilot. I remember the first week we were both in there [the NICU] and we were laughing and joking, because you just can't take it in. You live minute by minute. You are on survival mechanism. One of the nurses said to us that the first week is your honeymoon period, and we thought, "What do you mean, honeymoon?" Now we know. We didn't comprehend, until Bailey went.'

Facing the possibility of one's baby dying is, in some cases, crystallised by discussion of withdrawal of treatment being necessary. Rachel describes how she and her husband were called in to see the consultant to discuss whether to continue treatment and whether this 'would just prolong Emmy's pain and suffering or if it would help her. He didn't think it would help her.' Rachel recalls: 'I was devastated, but I couldn't give up on her.' When Michael was two weeks and four days old Debby and Martin were asked to discuss withdrawing life support from him. The problems that he had, which were themselves considerable, were being worsened by his need for assisted ventilation using high pressure and high oxygen concentrations. The suggestion by the medical team, as the only option left for him, was to try continuous positive airways pressure (CPAP) rather than fully assisted ventilation, to see if Michael could manage on this. This was thought unlikely to be successful and if Michael did not cope, it was suggested that assisted ventilation should not be resumed (Barrett 2007). Debby explains the factors which influenced their decision to try CPAP: 'If Michael was suffering then I wanted it to end, I did not want him to suffer any more than he had already. The thoughts of him dying slowly and painfully was more than I could deal with. I did not want him to live a life, trapped within a mind and body that did not work... I loved him enough to be able to let him go, to prevent him suffering for the rest of his life.' As well as her concerns for Michael, Debby recalls: 'My concern was not only for him but for his brothers, too. We always stated that we could cope with a child who had a certain level of disability, but thinking of his siblings I did not want to bring home a child that would have a major impact on their lives.' Amid all these considerations, Debby also remembers: 'We also wanted Michael to be able to make the decision for himself. I remember feeling that although I didn't want him suffering any more it would be so much easier if he decided that he'd had enough, and slipped away peacefully' (Barrett 2007). The decision was made to try CPAP, with the agreement that if this did not work for Michael, there would be no more intervention, and his short life would end.

Debby describes their feelings on the day when Michael was to be transferred to CPAP: 'The journey there [to the hospital] was difficult. Martin and I both with our own thoughts, but both of us realising that maybe the first time we would get to hold our son was as he died.' She continues: 'I was not totally convinced I could actually be with him as he died. I'd seen him a few days before when they changed his ventilator tube, and as the tube was removed he was terrified, I did not want my last memory of my son to be one of him panicking. I was not sure I would ever be able to sleep again, and that vision of him still haunts me even now almost seven years later' (Barrett 2007). Debby recalls how she and Martin sat in the parents room while Michael was switched to CPAP: 'I just could not cope with the thought of being there as my son was disconnected from the ventilator, so we sat in the parent's room, waiting for a call back to the unit or for them to appear in the doorway, so we could hold Michael as he passed. Time stopped.' Debby and Martin remained there for what seemed like 'for ever', before a nurse came to tell them Michael was coping on CPAP (Barrett 2007).

The response of Debby and Martin to Michael's initial survival indicates how hard it is for families to appreciate the implications of prematurity and critical illness unless these are very clearly explained, and the assumptions which can be made regarding their understanding. Debby and Martin went home, a burden lifted from them. Their baby had survived. Debby describes how far they were from realising that their understanding was incomplete: 'It wasn't until the next day, when one of our "favourite" nurses was talking to me about how she'd had to peep through the doors on her way in, to see if Michael was still there, because she hadn't expected him to be that it dawned on me. No one had expected him to survive the transfer and they certainly hadn't expected him to make it through the night. We had gone home thinking that because he survived the transfer we were home free' (Barrett 2007).

The Long Haul

Very often babies who are born extremely prematurely are in hospital for a very long time. Siobhan was in hospital for 81 days. Mollie came home after five months. Michael was 22 weeks and 5 days old when he came home, and Niamh was in hospital for four months. Chris describes: 'You don't realise how long it will be. The first week nothing sinks in, then the second week, things sink in, and then you've been there a month and then you start to think: "How long is this going to be?"'

The impossibility of ever knowing when the end of their baby's neo-natal stay was in sight was described by all their parents. Siobhan required assisted ventilation for approximately six weeks, and Evelyn recalls how she 'wondered if she would ever come off it'. She describes how Siobhan experienced 'ups and downs, collapsed lungs, aspirations, infections' before finally coming home. Chris explains: 'We found we could never look at targets. You just had to hope. You set targets and then missed them. With Mollie she was doing really well and then she was back on a ventilator. That was November. She was born in September, and in November she had just come off the ventilator and suddenly, again, it was touch and go if she was going to make it. This is two months down the line when you feel like things should have progressed. That was a reality check: after Bailey we were pinning all our hopes on Mollie and everything seemed to be going all right and then all of a sudden we were back to square one.' Rachel also describes the unstable times with Niamh and Emmy, with improvements followed by deteriorations in their conditions. Niamh initially did 'much better than was expected of a 25-weeker'. She weaned from high frequency oscillation ventilation within 24 hours, and progressed to CPAP at two weeks. However, from three weeks of age she deteriorated, required assisted ventilation to be resumed, and remained critically ill. An ultrasound revealed that she had large bleeds on both sides of her brain, and Rachel recalls, 'they weren't sure if she would ever walk, talk even breathe by herself'. Niamh deteriorated again, and was found to have candial septicaemia. Three weeks later her long line blocked and routine screening of the tip showed this to be the focus of infection. Three weeks later Niamh was back on CPAP and three days later on low-flow oxygen. She then developed osteomyelitis, recovered from this, and was finally able to go home two weeks later, four months after she was born. With Emmy, it was only after four months and two days, when she finally moved from the intensive care unit to her own room, that Rachel recalls: 'It really feels like we are on our way home now! I can't wait to get you home, I know anything could happen at any time but I am letting myself get a bit excited now!' (Dickinson 2007).

Michael also had many ups and downs during his long stay in the NICU and the special care baby unit (SCBU). This included a transfer to another hospital for ophthalmic evaluation of retinopathy of prematurity, for an echocardiogram, and to have his (extremely large) inguinal hernias surgically corrected. After his transfer, his respiratory effort, rate and oxygen requirements went up, and Debby describes: 'Suddenly, we found ourselves back in the level one high dependency unit, and back on a ventilator.' Michael spent two days in the high dependency unit, and 24 hours back on a ventilator. Debby recalls: 'It was awful, I was beside myself, I couldn't believe that we had come so far and here we were back on a ventilator' (Barrett 2007).

This ongoing inability to predict when progress will be sustained, and the steps forwards followed by steps backwards, mean that many parents begin their relationship with their baby with ongoing, day-to-day uncertainty about their health and even their survival.

Transitions

Another aspect of having a critically ill premature baby which many parents experience is moving from an intensive care to high dependency area or from the NICU to the SCBU. Although this is a positive sign that their baby's condition is improving, and the much hoped for end of the neo-natal long haul is in sight, the change in environment and level of supervision which babies have in a less intensive environment can be disquieting for parents. Debby recalls when Michael moved to the SCBU: 'Over the last ten weeks we had got so used to having more or less one-to-one nursing. In the SCBU there is roughly one nurse to four or more babies. It was, shall we say, a bit of a shock to the system' (Barrett 2007). Martin had been warned by a colleague about the difference between the NICU and the SCBU, but it was still unsettling. He explained: 'It can feel like they don't care, because there just aren't as many of them.' In addition, the level of monitoring which babies have outside the NICU is reduced. Although the monitoring equipment seen initially can be overwhelming and frightening for parents, its reduction may also be daunting. Chris explains: 'When we were in intensive care, we got used to the monitors, and when we moved out we were actually quite worried at first going into high dependency. But after she had been in high dependency for a while it was lovely, there wasn't so much noise, it was quieter, everyone was more relaxed.'

As well as the transition from the NICU to the SCBU, parents whose babies have been born prematurely have, at some stage, to move from neo-natal to general paediatric services. Like the transition from the NICU to the SCBU, this is a milestone, but one which again can be difficult. Tracy describes how she, Chris and Mollie became very familiar with and well-known at the neo-natal unit and the staff there before being transferred. 'At just over a year we were transferred to paediatrics, and that was quite traumatic actually. Because we knew the people and then we were just discharged to paediatrics. For a year we were with the SCBU, and I knew they were still at the end of the phone if I needed them, but really we had left. It was goodbye. They knew what had happened, they knew where we'd been, and you are suddenly with a stranger.'

Summary

When a baby is born extremely prematurely, the time that they spend in the NICU is likely to be long, and exhausting emotionally and physically for their parents.

Having an extremely premature baby means that parents often do not have the immediate contact that they would expect with their baby, and their newborn baby looks and inhabits an environment which is very different from that which is anticipated. The intensity of the neo-natal experience includes not only the physical environment, but parents seeing their baby suffer and being aware that they may not survive. The unpredictability of any progress which their baby makes means that parents can live for many weeks and months in timeless suspense, unable to hope, and reluctant to do so for fear of their hopes being dashed.

As well as the intensity of the environment and experience of having a critically ill premature baby, parents may be unable to spend as much time as they would want to with their baby, whom may be some distance from the family home. This can mean that other family members, for example siblings and grandparents, as well as parents, do not have the experience which they expected with the newborn baby. It also means that parents may be cut off from support from families and friends by distance and by others being uncertain of how to respond to their new arrival.

The parents of premature babies have a great deal to take in, and this means that healthcare staff may have to be very clear, but compassionate, in what they say; they must check parents' comprehension of this and be aware that the enormity of the situation may be too much for them to fully absorb. The times when their baby moves from the NICU to the SCBU and from neo-natal to paediatric services can also be daunting for parents, and those supporting them should be aware of this.

Chapter 5

Families whose Children have Complex Needs

A child having complex and continuing health needs has the potential to affect the whole family. This includes parents, siblings and their extended family. The care and support which these children receive should therefore be seen in the context of its effect on and assistance to the child and their family, rather than just the child. Doing this includes taking into account relationships between family members, changes to the family home, family outings, holidays, and the effects which having a brother or sister with complex and continuing health needs may have on siblings.

Some of the effects of the children's needs on their families, which parents and siblings have described, are discussed in this chapter.

Relationships

Having a child with complex and continuing health needs can affect the relationship between their parents. Chapter 3 describes how parents whose children have complex and continuing health needs often have very little time for themselves. This means that the time which they have to spend with one another and the quality of this time is often very limited, as Rosemary describes: 'You never ever get time to yourself. When you do get "time for me" all you want to do is sleep. We are lucky that we have another sitting room (away from Hollie and Christian's sitting room and the room which the care staff use), but both Colin and I rarely get a chance to sit down together in the other room, and even then we're too busy watching what's going on with Hollie and Christian, so you have very little time together. When we do get time together a lot of discussion is about the practicalities of care, not the children themselves. The main topic of conversation is care. I have heard that many marriages split up, and I'm not surprised because you have no time to yourselves.' Helen also explains: 'Looking back [to Ryan's early years] it was in some ways a real strain on the marriage. At times it brought us closer together, but there were times when John came in from work, after maybe an 11-hour day, and I'd say, "The nurse had gone off sick and one of us has to stay up all night", and we both had to go to work the next day.' In some cases the child or children's needs are too great for one parent, and the relationship ends. When Sophia was diagnosed with congenital central hypoventilation syndrome Cheryl's husband left, because he felt unable to cope with this. Cheryl has therefore had to cope with Zak and Sophia's day-to-day care alone, with support from her parents. As well as the effect which having a child with complex needs may have on existing relationships, Alison explains how parents who are managing their child's care alone also need time to form new relationships: 'I am on my own. I've been in a relationship a year and we need that time.'

As well as a lack of time alone together, parents often have few opportunities to socialise together. For example, Val explains that, unless the family has respite care they never go out together: 'At New Year I went to the beginning of a party and my husband went to the second half.'

The Family Home

A child with complex and continuing health needs often requires changes to be made to the family home, which can affect the whole family. The amount of space required to store equipment is often considerable: Catherine's supplies occupy half of the garage, and Cheryl and Steve have had to find space for Hannah's corner seat, her comfy seat, her wheelchair and her standing frame in their dining room. Hannah also has a bath frame, which has to be removed to enable them to bath Philipa, and Cheryl is aware that one day they will also need a hoist or, they hope, a purpose built wet room adaptation instead. As well as the space required, the equipment which children need may alter the home environment in other ways. Michael uses an oxygen concentrator, which is the size of a small fridge, is very noisy, and blows out hot air. Debby describes how the family have had to 'get used to it, it is like living by a major road'.

As well as equipment, families may have to adapt their homes to accommodate their child's needs. The Hethringtons have had to have a hoist and the rails for this fitted throughout their house, a lift put in to take Lucy upstairs, the bathroom redesigned to accommodate hoisting equipment and to ensure Lucy's safety, the kitchen rebuilt so that she has access to this and to the upstairs of the house and so that they have space to store everything which she needs. These alterations have required the house to be almost completely redesigned. Because the changes were largely dictated by those assisting with the funding, and by Lucy's needs, the Hethringtons had very little choice in what was done to their own home. They no longer have space for things that were of huge sentimental value, and it is not the home which they chose. Mrs Hethrington explains: 'I liked my house as it was. There was nothing wrong with it. I liked how it was before.' In addition, managing the construction work on the house was difficult, in particularly as there was no option but for Lucy, who is prone to respiratory infections, to be there while the work was done. Mrs Hethrington explains: 'They couldn't do all the work every day because of the dust, for Lucy's chest. We had building work going on with a suction machine in the middle.'

If a child has behavioural problems, these can also affect the home environment. Once Michael was able to remove his clothes he developed a preference for being naked, and as he was not potty trained he also started smearing. Debby describes how she would go to the toilet and come back to find the windows and the TV covered in faeces. 'One morning I went upstairs to get school clothes for his older brother and by the time I got down stairs Michael had left a trail all over the downstairs of the house, having ridden a push-bike through it' (Barrett 2007). As he got older and more mobile, 'all ornaments were thrown from window ledges, the bookcase emptied, video cases shredded, drawers emptied, and DVDs, Playstation games, and so on chewed. He drew on the walls, he tore wallpaper, he chewed jigsaws and books. It is heart-breaking to find objects of sentimental value in pieces when you think they are out of reach. I don't think I can stress how disheartening this whole phase of his life was, it is hard to see your child destroying your environment, the home you have worked hard to build' (Barrett 2007).

In some cases, families have to move home because of their child's needs. Cheryl and Steve have moved twice. The first time, from a small terraced house, both because of the size and nature of the house and because the medical and support services for Hannah in that borough were poor. It then became apparent that Hannah would not be able to walk. Their new house had stairs and four steps up to the front door, so the family moved again, to a bungalow. Cheryl describes how 'we would never have bought a bungalow ordinarily, and obviously with my wage gone, we have had to push ourselves. It has been the best move possible for us. But again it's something we'd never have done.'

Family Activities

Families often describe how they strive to prevent their child's needs from altering their lives. Sharon explains: 'We are of the opinion that we will carry on our lives as normal as far as possible, so that Zoë fits in with us.' However, despite these intentions, Sharon reports, 'it impacts on everything. It is the little things, which when you put them all together, it's a lot that other people take for granted.'

Although families often continue to go on outings, these have to be planned more meticulously than would otherwise be the case, and always with the child's specific needs in mind. This is partly because of a lack of facilities for disabled children hampering the whole family enjoying days out together and limiting the venues that they can visit. Sharon explains: 'If you've got siblings you don't always want to home in on special needs all the time. You want to try and integrate with everyone else, but often you can't do it.' In addition, the planning which a child's needs necessitate often limits the spontaneity of outings. Sharon explains: 'If we want to go to the beach you can't just tell Zoë to get her swimming costume, get in the car, we'll get something to eat there.' Sharon has to ensure that Zoë has everything she needs, including her wheelchair, whatever she will need to eat, appropriate cutlery to eat this with, consider if the place where they are going will be wheelchair friendly, and as one cannot take a wheelchair on the sand, how Zoë will get across the beach, whether there is something for her to play with on the beach, and how she will spend her time because she cannot be easily transported from the sand to the sea. In addition, when children have complex and continuing health needs it often means that for them to go out with their siblings two adults need to be present, which restricts the occasions on which this can happen.

Family celebrations are also sometimes affected by children's needs. This may be because the family cannot be together. For example, Debby describes how Michael has a 'habit' of being in hospital for Christmas and birthdays. Of Michael's first Christmas at home (aged five) Debby recalls: 'It was lovely waking up on Christmas morning as a family. I cannot describe how wonderful it was to wake on Christmas morning and have all my children there, opening their Christmas presents, being together as a complete family and not having one member missing' (Barrett 2007).

A child with complex and continuing health needs may mean that the roles which other members of the family take on, or their relationships with the child, are different from their expectations. For example, Helen describes how visits to close relatives may be more restricted than one would expect. She recalls the significance of the first time she took David to his nanny's: 'She had been to the hospital and she would pop to our house, but to actually be able to go to her…we couldn't go round with all the equipment at first, but once we got David into a routine and he had slept for a couple of hours we could then go.' Cheryl also explains how Zak's illness affected his grandparents' early relationship with him. Zak was in hospital in Stoke for the first nine months of his life, and Cheryl's parents went from Manchester to visit him at weekends. He was their only grandchild and they 'felt they were missing out'.

Holidays

The needs which children have, or the provision for these, means that families are often restricted in their holiday options. Jo describes trying to organise holidays for the whole family as 'a nightmare'. If Mitchell accompanies the family on holiday, they need a member of staff to provide his night care. Their primary care trust will only fund night care if this is in the family home, so Jo's family has to pay for this when they take Mitchell on holiday. As the carers can only work a certain number of nights, for one week's holiday Mitchell needs at least two staff, and thus the family has at least two sets of travel costs to meet. This makes the cost of any holiday very high: a recent one-week visit to Jo's parents cost £1000 for Mitchell's care. This restriction on funding is not universal and Helen recalls, 'the health authority did always fund a nurse to come on holiday with us, and they would fund her accommodation and travel'.

As well as funding issues, having to be accompanied by staff affects when holidays can be taken. Mitchell needs to be cared for by people who know him, and are trained to meet his needs, so holidays have to be taken when such staff are available to accompany the family. In addition, having staff with the family, while necessary, can be intrusive. Mitchell's family needs to provide and extra room for the carer and, because the staff provide night cover, the family have to be quiet during the day because the staff are asleep. Staying in is therefore not really an option, and, given the complexities of taking Mitchell out all day every day, this is also problematic. The intrusion which staff constitute on a family holiday is one reason why David's family chose to stop taking staff on family holidays. Helen explains: 'After a while it got so that we just thought: this isn't our family holiday. So now we just manage without and muddle through.'

The type of holiday accommodation which families need also requires careful consideration. Sharon explains that this includes precise details, such as: 'What kind of floors it has got, because if it is stone floors Zoë's going to go flying, and if it has mats everywhere, if you step on one of those you'll go flying if you're not careful, and if you're bunny hopping everywhere, or using a walker, because she doesn't use her wheelchair indoors, its not suitable. And is it literally all on one level, or has it got little steps down? We've been away before and they say: "It's all on one level" but it's got little steps.' Cheryl also has to consider minute details when she books holiday accommodation for Zak and Sophia. This includes how many plug points their rooms have and where they are, to make certain that they will be near enough to the children's beds to facilitate overnight assisted ventilation.

The amount of equipment and supplies that their children need is another factor which parents have to consider when they go on holiday. Val describes one such occasion: 'I didn't go to bed until midnight for about three nights before we went away (for a week, within the UK). I do have checklists, because I need those for overnight respite, but you need however many times as much.' Some idea of the amount of extra luggage which the family may need to take on holiday, simply because of their child's additional needs, is illustrated by Debby's list of what Michael needs for a five-day trip away:

- three ZH size 02 cylinders (2400 litres)
- one nasal cannula and face tape
- twenty-one x 500 ml bottles of Tentrini
- five x 1000 ml flexitainer feed bottles
- five tubes to fit the bottles
- two extension sets
- five kangaroo giving sets
- feed pump
- stand for feed pump
- nine x 10 ml syringes
- one spare Mickey button for the GPEG
- one tube KY jelly
- one x 300 ml tube of vitaquick (feed thickener)
- one x 100 ml bottle of Klaricid
- one x 300 ml bottle of zantac
- one x 200 ml bottle of domperidone
- one packet of nappies
- baby wipes
- bottle opener
- blue syringe adapters
- extra clothes to cover for vomiting episodes
- telephone numbers of medical professionals
- small background history just in case.

Val recalls when the family went to Spain: 'We had to take all Catherine's feeds and two [feed] pumps in case one failed, one in our hand luggage. They did give us extra luggage allowance for the bottles of milk. I spoke to this guy at the airline and he said if you can weigh the milk we can give you extra luggage allowance, so I got the bathroom scales and I was piling all this milk up and perched the pump on the top.'

Obtaining the additional supplies needed for holidays can sometimes be difficult. Val requested enough of the sterile water needed for Catherine's gastrojejunostomy feeds to last for a one-week holiday (Saturday to Saturday). The sterile water was not provided until the Friday, which made planning and packing very difficult. Even then, only exactly one week's supply was provided, leaving no supply for the final Saturday of their holiday and the Sunday before services resumed on the Monday. This meant that Val had the task of seeking alternatives in addition to the already immense planning required for the holiday.

As well as the equipment and supplies which Michael needs, the liaison required to make trips away from home as safe as possible is a further task which Debby has to take on. The community nurses from Michael's home town usually contact the community nurses in the town where the family are visiting to ensure that they are aware of Michael's needs. While this support is very useful, it is another point which other families do not have to consider when planning short breaks.

When families go abroad, their planning has to include in-flight practicalities. Sharon explains: 'You've got to get Zoë on the aeroplane, make sure the wheelchair arrives in one piece, which isn't all that easy, think about the flight: have I got food for her and how will she eat what we've got on the plane, then at the time [when the family went to the USA] she couldn't sit in a plane seat, so we had to take a car seat, so by the time you've done that, and made sure you've got all her medication, and everything else, you think "Was it really worth it?" You're absolutely shattered.' Sharon also recalls how she was almost prevented from taking Zoë's special cutlery on the flight to the USA, because it presented a security risk. She explains, 'I'd put her cutlery in my bag, because it's special shaped cutlery. I said, "But I can't feed her any other way on the plane." I was asked "What do you mean?" I said, "Well, she can't use a plastic knife and fork. She can't go on a 13-hour flight with no food. Look at it. It's as blunt as anything. You can tell she's disabled. She's in a wheelchair." Eventually they let me get on with it.' Val also describes some of the practical security considerations which she has to take into account for flights: 'I had to ask the consultant to write to the airline so that we could take the syringes and drugs.'

The need for in-flight planning to include every eventuality was illustrated when Sophia fell asleep on a return journey from the USA, requiring

Cheryl to institute assisted ventilation in the aeroplane. Even with detailed planning for such an event, space in an aircraft is an issue, despite Cheryl and her children having upgraded to first class to maximise the space which they had. Cheryl describes how 'we had to have her lying on the floor in the aisle, and it was amazing how many people wanted to use the toilet on that flight'.

The amount of assistance that families will need to embark and disembark from flights also has to be considered. When Cheryl took Zak and Sophia to the USA, she spent countless hours arranging the family's flights and ensuring that they would have assistance at each end to take the equipment that the children need on and off the aircraft. This was provided at Manchester Airport; however, on arrival in the USA Cheryl recalls, 'there was no help and we couldn't get off without someone helping us with our equipment. Eventually, the carer who was with us just said: "Right kids, put your seatbelts on, we're going home."' After an hour or so of waiting, the family were finally given assistance, but only because of their refusal to move without it.

Where children are oxygen-dependent, taking them on holiday includes the complexity of organising oxygen supplies and funding this. If families are thinking of going abroad, the arrangements for in-flight and at-destination oxygen often make this impractical and too costly to even contemplate. Rachel explains: 'I'd love to take them abroad. We can get oxygen in the USA, but Emmy would need oxygen on the plane because of pressure changes, and they want £200 each way for in-flight oxygen, and £2000 for oxygen over there.' Even within the UK, needing oxygen limits families' holiday options. Rachel describes her recent attempts to book a family holiday in a caravan: 'The lady was really good, and then I rang her a couple of weeks ago and asked her about the oxygen and she said, "Oh, I didn't know about that. You can't keep that in the caravan." But then she said she had a chalet we could have instead so I said, "All right then." Then she must have had doubts about it and she sent me an email saying that she was sorry but she couldn't accept the liability. So she cancelled our holiday.'

If families need to hire a car, this can create further issues. Cheryl found that Hannah's needs meant that the type of car seat she requires differs from EU standards. This meant that her seat for their holiday car in Menorca could not be booked in advance from the UK. Cheryl was told that they could alter the car seat, which they had to book when they arrived, and in the event this was no problem, but it left an element of uncertainty over the holiday arrangements. Sharon also explains that hiring a car is more costly than it would be for another family with two children: 'It pushes the price up because you've got to get a car that's big enough to take a wheelchair. You can't take Zoë's electric wheelchair because that would just put the price up too much, but you've got to get something that's big enough to take a manual chair.'

Travel insurance can also be a challenge to organise, and costly. Cheryl and Steve can only insure Hannah via Epilepsy Action. Cheryl estimates that the cost of Zak and Sophia's insurance for two weeks in the USA was in the region of £1000 and Rachel was told that Emmy's insurance for travel to the USA would cost £2000.

These factors all mean that organising and going on holiday as a family can present a huge challenge. However, if families choose to take a holiday without their child, they have to arrange alternative care for them. If Jo and Stan want to take Daniel abroad, they have to organise care for Mitchell, and, given the funding problems for out-of-home care, this means arranging for someone else to stay in their home to care for Mitchell there. Last year Jo, Stan and Daniel went to Spain, the first holiday abroad that they had taken together, and Jo's parents looked after Mitchell. However, the family do not feel able to ask them to do that again, so this year they will be unable to take a family holiday abroad. At present, Jo's family only go to her parents for holidays, because the cost and organisational issues would be too much to go elsewhere. Like Jo, Debby and Martin usually now stay with 'relatives who are used to the amount of equipment we come with' for their holidays.

Finances

Changes in parents' ability to engage in paid employment often mean that families have a significant change in their financial status. For example, Alison explains: 'I was financially secure before I had Peter. I had my own house, I had a job. I sold my other house and moved here where I am a bit nearer my parents. Although I was financially secure, things have become very tight.' Mr Hethrington also recounts how, as Lucy has become older and more dependent, 'what money we did have put by is gone'. Although the family was never affluent, looking back to when he and his wife could work, Mr Hethrington recalls, 'we were comfortable then'.

In addition to the loss of income, Sharon explains that everything costs more for a child with complex needs. This includes basic items, such as toys: 'Going out and buying Zoë a pram for her doll. It's: is it the right height for her? The right weight that if she leans on it she won't go flying? Can she use it? You don't just go out and buy toys, they've got to be practical. That adds to the cost.' Cheryl and Steve also explain how 'we never ever thought we'd see Hannah on a bike, then we tried her on this trike [at a display], and we were both in tears watching her, and we said "Whatever it takes she's having one." Then we found it was £800 and was "She's still having one, but it might take time."' Fortunately, Steve's father, uncles and aunts organised a fundraising event so that the tricycle could be purchased for Hannah, but this illustrates the difference in the cost and thought which has to go into obtaining toys and other play equipment for children who have complex and continuing health needs.

As described previously, families may have to make adaptations to their housing to accommodate their child's needs, and these are another source of expense. Trevor and Sharon had to remortgage their house two years ago, in order to have a bedroom and bathroom built downstairs because Zoë is unable to manage stairs and was becoming too heavy to carry up and down. Alison also explains how many incidental expenses parents can incur because of their child's needs: 'If you want to travel anywhere, you have to hire a larger vehicle as these children [with congenital central hypoventilation syndrome) do not qualify for a disability car despite all their equipment and the need for a vehicle to be on hand.' As Alison notes, there are schemes which enable families to obtain some discounts, for example on the cost of having to run a ventilator every night, but these are often not well known and families are not routinely made aware of them. Alison describes how 'you find out as you go along. You just find out. So by word of mouth I've spread the word about that'.

As well as the availability of information on the existence of schemes to provide financial assistance or benefits, the assistance which is available to families is not always easy to access. Alison explains how 'You need a very good social worker to go through all the complicated benefits forms. They are horrific. You're in a state of stress and to be faced with that as well is horrendous.' Alison describes how the stress associated with the financial side of having a child with complex and continuing health needs as something which is often played down: 'I have heard of, and I have seen myself, relationships that break down and people in financial trouble, and it is a big source of stress which is underplayed.'

Siblings

In most cases, children's siblings appear to be very close to them, for example Judy explains that Simon has a 'fantastic relationship' with his middle brother, Paul. Debby also describes how her other children 'just see Michael as himself. They just incorporate Michael into their lives.'

Having a brother or sister who has complex and continuing health needs can, nonetheless, have an effect on siblings, which includes positive points. Daniel describes the advantages of being Mitchell's brother, such as receiving double shares of advent calendar chocolate and Easter eggs, as people give these to Mitchell without realising that he cannot eat. He also feels that he has gained more friends through Mitchell because the staff who provide evening care for Mitchell often become 'sort of friends'. He can go to Mitchell's room and talk to and play with them, so being Mitchell's brother gives him more options for things to do and people to socialise with in the evenings. The reverse of this is that, for some children, having care staff in their home can intrude on their lives. William explains that the way in which his family's home is now designed means that staff being present is no great inconvenience. However, before the family moved to their present home the staff had to sit in the lounge. This could be awkward, because of 'having a stranger in our family lounge'. Helen also describes how different service providers have very different attitudes towards siblings. She reports that before the hospice took over the management of David's support, staff would exclude William from his brother's life and even from areas of his own home. For example, if he got up early and went to David's room before Helen did the nurse would ask him to leave the room as she was not responsible for him, only David. Helen explains: 'Just think what must have gone through William's mind. He would walk into the lounge or David's bedroom at 7am, a nurse was playing games with David, and William, who was only three at the time, would want to join in. He was then asked to leave the room, in his own house.' The family spoke to the team manager about this and were told that unfortunately this was how it had to be because the nurse was paid to look after David, not William. This attitude to siblings changed completely when the hospice took over providing the care staff for David, to the extent that if Helen and John wanted to go out on some occasions, the carer could look after William as well.

Although they may themselves be very close to their brother or sister, siblings may have to respond to or cope with their peers' responses to their brother or sister. In some cases, this is not a problem or issue. Daniel's peers appear to be as untroubled by Mitchell as Daniel is, and 'don't say much' about him. William also reports that, although his peers noticed David having some additional needs, their comments were never negative. However, it is something that most parents are aware of as a potential problem. Sharon describes how Amy 'had a friend, a few years ago now, who said "Your sister's not normal, she's bunny-hopping everywhere. She must be a bunny rabbit." And Amy said, "my sister can't help it, she's got cerebral palsy" and I didn't know what to do, whether to tell her off or laugh, and in the end I left it, and thought, no she'd dealt with it in her way.' Debby also notes that although her children have no problems with Michael 'James has had some difficulties with people teasing him about Michael's special needs, which he has found hard to deal with, and one of James' friends excludes Michael when he comes over'.

Having a child who has complex and continuing health needs can also reduce the time which their parents can spend with their other children. Rachel describes how each of her children's' needs affect the others: 'Niamh needs time, and I feel sorry for her because I haven't always got time, because of Emmy, I'm not spending the time I want to with Niamh.' Cheryl also explains that Sophia being in Stoke for six months when Zak was three and a half years old has had an effect on him: 'Even now, he is a lot more clingy than Sophia is. If Sophia's not well he asks me will I be there when he comes home. He's worried all the time, and if I call the school in the morning and say that Sophia isn't coming to school he'll be asking all the time if I'll be there when he comes home from school. I'll say to him "Why do you think I might not be there?" And he'll say, "Because Sophia's ill." He knows she might be in hospital and I might not be there.' William also recalls his parents sometimes having to go to hospital with David during the night. However, while he recalls, 'it was quite weird waking up and finding just Nan there and no Mum and Dad', he does not see this in a negative light. He explains that as David was in hospital for a year or so when he was two to three years old, 'that's the way it was. I didn't know any different'.

The activities which siblings of children with complex needs can participate in can be affected by their brother or sister's needs. Although this may not be problematic for their children, it is often something that their parents are very aware of. William recalls: 'Early on, Mum and Dad were very conscious of David's needs, and made sure they treated us equally. They would take me to places and treat me a lot.' Siblings can, nonetheless, miss out on day-to-day events because of their brother or sister's needs. Lucy's older brother, Ryan used to love going out on his motorbike with his father, but this eventually became impossible because his father could not leave Lucy. In addition, because of a lack of provision for disabled children in many places, incorporating a child who has a disability and their siblings in activities can be a challenge. Sharon explains: 'I've had Amy say "I'd like to go to Paultons Park" or "I'd like to go to the pictures" and I'm thinking "How am I going to do that?" and what's the point of going to Paulton's Park when we can't get Zoë on half the rides, because we've got to pick her up to go on rides and she's getting heavy to pick up and she won't enjoy the rides, and not all of it's wheelchair friendly. Amy wants to do things as a family, or even just with her Mum and Dad, and unless we get Zoë looked after we can't both go, so it's a case of trying to balance things, and not always saying "We can't do that because of your sister." Bless her heart, Amy never complains. But I am very aware that I sometimes have to say "We can't do that because of your sister," "We can't do that I'm too tired," "We can't take your sister there." And it's almost like she's on the back seat and we can only do things Zoë can do. For instance, she asked on her birthday "Can we go out and eat in so and so?" and I'm thinking "Hmm, I can't get Zoë's wheelchair in there and there's nothing in there that's going to be suitable for her to eat." So it's a case of "Well, can we go to this place instead" and it's "Yeah, if we have to Mum." And she accepts it all.'

Their parents' availability because of one of their brother's or sister's needs can also mean that a child's everyday activities are restricted as Sharon explains: 'Because Amy and Zoë's Dad's away a lot it's, "Oh Mum I want to go out and can you come and pick me up?" And it's, "Well I can't because your sister will be in bed." Most ten-year-olds might not be in bed at half-past seven but Zoë is, because she gets very very tired.' Parents' exhaustion from meeting their child's needs, as much as the needs themselves, can also affect siblings' activities. For example, Val explains: 'Thomas used to do Tae Kwon Do, and he did really well in that and got to black belt and then he gave up, but I think it was just as much me that gave up on it because it was just exhausting taking them both out twice a week after school.'

Parents often describe their other children as very mature for their age. This may be partly because they have had to face issues related to their sibling's health which other children do not, including the possibility of their brother or sister's death. Rachel explains that if she has to stay overnight in hospital with Emmy, 'the other girls think Emmy will die, because that [when she was initially in hospital, in the NICU] was the worst time in her life and they thought she was going to die'. It may also be because of the roles and responsibilities which they have had to take on related to their siblings' needs. Sharon explains: 'I think Amy's had to grow up a lot more quickly than other children her age, because I've only got one pair of hands and there are things she can help me do.' Rachel also describes Jodie as, 'So mature for her age and I feel so sorry for her. She is the one that has had to help me.'

As well as taking responsibility for giving their parents practical assistance, siblings often have a greater sense of responsibility for their brother or sister than other children might. Even when she is away from home, Jodie seems to feel responsible for checking on her sisters' well-being. Rachel explains what happened when Jodie was on holiday with a friend: 'Every time she rings she says "Are they all OK?" and I say, "Yes, they're OK" and she says, "Can I speak to them?" and she's not daft, if I said she can't speak to them she'd want to know why, what had gone wrong.' Although he does not describe himself as taking on additional responsibilities as a child, William appears to have taken some responsibility for enabling his parents to get breaks from David's care. David used to go to a hospice for respite care. However, there came a point at which he did not want to go, but without this respite care William and David's parents did not get a break. William describes how he began to go with him and stay in the family room. Although he recalls having fun with the other children and the staff and 'ended up being more like staff' this represents a difference in his life, and a way in which children may be aware of their parents' workload and, often unconsciously, take on some responsibility for reducing this.

As they get older, siblings may take on more responsibilities. William describes how as he got older and now, during times when he is at home from university, he can volunteer to supervise David so that his parents can go out. He is also aware that being David's brother has implications for his own future. While he knows that his parents will do their best to look after David, there are long-term issues for him, including whether David's current support from the National Health Service will continue and how this will be arranged. William explains that while he will be 'quite happy to step in and take full responsibility, it is a lot of responsibility'. The possibility of him taking on responsibility for his brother means that William has to consider how he will manage if he has a full-time job, and where David will live, 'with me, right next to me, how will care be sorted out?' As William explains, there are not many children with David's condition that are older than him, so he and his brother, and how support will be organised, is very much untested ground for service provision. William stresses that he is prepared to accept this responsibility, and his girlfriend (of three years) understands this responsibility. It is, nonetheless, a consideration which not all university graduates have to add to decision-making about their futures.

Summary

A child with complex and continuing health needs can have effects on all the members of their family, including parents, siblings and their extended family.

Parents may have less time to spend with their partner, and this time may be primarily devoted to discussing their child's needs and the arrangements for their care rather than to developing their relationship. The child's needs may also mean that significant changes occur in the family home, including some families needing to move. A child with complex and continuing health needs can also affect the ease with which family outings can be arranged, the locations which families can use, the holidays which families take, and the amount of planning which these activities require. The child's needs may also alter their family's financial status, because of loss of parental earnings and because many of the items which are suitable for children with complex needs are more expensive than equivalent items for children who do not have their needs.

Siblings' lives are often affected by their brother's or sister's needs. This includes additional responsibilities which they may take on, albeit often almost subconsciously, the time which their parents have to spend with them, and their ability to engage in leisure time or out of school activities. Siblings may also have to deal with their own awareness of their brother's or sister's condition and the risk which this poses to their ongoing health, and the responses which their peers have to their sibling. Despite this, as well as the challenges of having a sibling with complex and continuing health needs, positive aspects of this situation have been highlighted. Having a sibling with complex and continuing health needs does, none-theless, present siblings with considerations for their future which their peers may not have.

Chapter 6

Diagnosis

For some children who have complex and continuing health needs, a clear diagnosis is possible, and rapidly expedited. However, for many children the process of obtaining a diagnosis for their problems is a long and unclear road. The child and the family, not the child's diagnostic label, should always be the focus in providing care or support. However, because of the benefits and challenges which this can present for the child and their family, this chapter describes some of the experiences of children and their families in relation to diagnosis and the issues which seeking and having a diagnosis of the child's problems can present.

Problems with Diagnosis

In some cases, diagnosis of the cause of a child's problem or problems is difficult because the child has a variant of a disorder which not all professionals are aware of. For example, Hannah has an unusual variant of Rett syndrome which delayed her diagnosis. Cheryl explains how one consultant who saw her thought that she, 'looked like she had Rett, because she was so beautiful, but the tests were negative, and her epilepsy [atypically for Rett syndrome] had started so early'. Hannah had numerous investigations which did not provide an answer. Eventually a geneticist sent a sample of Hannah's blood for testing to a research project on girls who had a variant of Rett syndrome and Hannah's diagnosis was confirmed.

In other instances diagnosis is problematic because the disorder which the child has is rare and not widely known among professionals. For example, the staff at David's local hospital were unable to identify the cause of his problems and Helen recalls, 'for the first two weeks they didn't know what was wrong with him. They said: "He can't manage without the ventilator, but he can't be ventilated for ever." David was sent to a specialist hospital in London where congenital central hypoventilation syndrome was diagnosed.

Sometimes diagnosis is problematic because the child's problems do not exactly match any particular disorder. In Hollie and Christian's cases, the diagnosis of Kohlschutter syndrome was made after a long period of investigation and is still only that which most closely matches their presentation, not an absolute or clear-cut diagnosis. Rosemary explains that this is not through any fault of the staff involved: 'The tests that they did and the attitude at Great Ormond Street were excellent. They were really, really thorough. They searched every single avenue, tested every single area, and they couldn't have been more perfect. Eventually we saw a professor who was really good and I kept saying to him that a part of their genetics can be traced back to their teeth, because they've got no enamel on their teeth, either of them. He didn't let this go and he searched for years and eventually came up with Kohlschutter syndrome.'

In other cases it may be that diagnosis is delayed because the child is too young for their symptoms to be clear enough for a definitive diagnosis to be given. Sharon describes how Zoë did not initially have any major problems, and Sharon 'just thought she was a bit of an awkward baby'. When she was six months old the health visitor referred Zoë for some physiotherapy and Sharon saw a paediatrician who 'said he was 90 per cent sure she didn't have cerebral palsy, she was just a bit slow. Carry on with the physio.' When she was a year old Zoë was seen again, 'and basically he said, "Yes, she's got cerebral palsy."'

In some instances, diagnosis or identification of the extent of a problem may be delayed because healthcare professionals do not see any benefit in knowing this. Catherine was about three years old before the family became aware of the extent of her problems, and there was some reluctance on the part of medical staff to explore the cause of these. Val recalls how, when it became clear that Catherine was not progressing as one would expect, she asked the paediatrician if a magnetic resonance imaging (MRI) scan of Catherine's brain could be arranged. The response which she received was unexpected: 'The doctor said, "You may not find it very helpful: a scan will only show the anatomy of the brain it will not tell you how she will be affected functionally."' When Val explained that she wanted to know, if possible, the extent and nature of the damage, the doctor replied: 'You will only find out her functional ability as you go along.' Val describes his response as 'absolutely unbelievable. I suppose from his point of view it's expensive, there's a waiting list, and we know she has brain damage…but as a parent you want to know the cause, the extent, what it means, is it progressive?'

Some parents report that delays in diagnosis can occur because professionals are attached to the child and may themselves be reluctant to accept that a problem exists. Evelyn recalls how, in retrospect, it seems that Siobhan's paediatrician was unwilling to acknowledge the cause of her problems: 'I would say to him, when Siobhan was meant to be hitting her milestones, that I was worried. But he just kept reassuring me.' Evelyn explains: 'I'm not bitter with him. I don't think he actually wanted to admit to himself even that she had cerebral palsy. He looked after her fantastically.'

Listening to Parents

In some cases it appears that diagnosis is delayed because medical staff do not listen to parents or take note of their observations of their child. As well as having Rett syndrome, Lucy had craniostenosis. Mrs Hethrington recalls that she noticed early on that Lucy's head was an unusual shape, then, 'there was a thing on TV about craniostenosis. A friend saw it and called me to say "There's a girl on telly with a head like your Lucy's."' When Mrs Hethrington asked her GP about it, his response was that he had never heard of it and 'don't listen to what you hear on TV'. However, Mrs Hethrington took Lucy to see a paediatrician, 'who told me to go out and get a job' suggesting that Mrs Hethrington was worrying about Lucy's head because she had nothing else to do. The paediatrician also told Mrs Hethrington that this type of over-anxiety was 'quite common with a first child'. Lucy is Mrs Hethrington's second child. Mrs Hethrington obtained more information on craniostenosis, contacted the plastic surgery department at St James' Hospital, Leeds, and arranged for Lucy to be seen there. She explains that, at the appointment, the consultant 'just looked at her head and said "Definitely."' Mrs Hethrington explains, 'I knew she didn't look right. Yes, she looked pretty in pink but I was looking at her head from the top, every day, when she was in a buggy, and you could see her head was the wrong shape. The paediatrician just looked at her from the front and said she'd got a squint. But I could see her head was the wrong shape.'

Debby and Martin have experienced many challenges with Michael's diagnoses. Possibly the most traumatic was the way in which the diagnosis of autistic spectrum disorder was handled and the refusal of one professional in particular to listen to Debby. When he was two and a half, the community paediatrician diagnosed Michael as having attention deficit hyperactivity disorder (ADHD) and suggested treating him with ritalin. However, on Debby's insistence, Michael was referred to a specialist centre for neuro development assessment and to a neurologist. The neurologist described Michael as having 'autistic tendencies'. At the same time, Michael's behaviour was becoming increasingly difficult, and Debby's health visitor suggested a referral to the Child and Adolescent Mental Health Service (CAMHS) for advice on behaviour management. The consultation did nothing to clarify the diagnostic picture or to assist Debby to manage Michael's behaviour. Debby explains: 'The long and the short of it is that it didn't matter what I said, nor how many times I said it, the therapist was not listening. She was not prepared to take into account Michael's prematurity nor any of the things that he had experienced while growing and developing. It didn't count, except in the way it affected me, and my depression, and therefore how this affected my relationship with Michael. Michael's issues were to do with me, and my depression, and if I were not depressed then Michael would be fine. When I mentioned Michael's developmental delay, I was told that unless I "treated Michael like a normal three-year-old he would never be a normal three-year-old". When I questioned how that worked when he didn't have the understanding of a "normal" three-year-old, the reply was that he never would unless I treated him as such.' Debby continues: 'When I left there I hit rock bottom. I was devastated and reeled for weeks over the session that we'd had at the CAMHS, to the point where I seriously considered handing Michael over to Social Services, because it was obviously my relationship with him that was the problem' (Barrett 2007). Three months later Debby had the planned appointment with the neurodevelopment team and Michael was diagnosed as having autistic spectrum disorder.

In some cases, parents recall their own intuition and knowledge of their child making clear that a problem existed, even when the medical evidence was not absolutely clear or when this was dismissed by professionals. Evelyn describes how she always knew that something was wrong with Siobhan and how, when the diagnosis of cerebral palsy was made, she already knew. 'One time when we saw the paediatrician, I met a woman who had twins and one of them had cerebral palsy. I asked her what was wrong and she said it was cerebral palsy and I just looked at them and I thought, "Siobhan has that." I don't know why, just gut instinct. I had researched a lot about cerebral palsy on the internet, so when they actually told me, it just wasn't a shock. Everyone kept coming up to me and saying: "Are you OK, are you going to be OK, do you need to speak to someone?" But without anyone telling me I sort of, deep down, knew. I had hoped it wasn't, but I did know. I suppose just a mother's instinct. Especially when you've had a baby, and they're not crawling at eight months. You put a couple of months down to catching up from being premature, but you just know there's a problem.'

Realising the Extent of the Problem

Although, in some cases, parents are aware very early on that their child has a problem, in others the problem, or the reality and severity of this, can become apparent very slowly. This sometimes happens because other events mask the problem, for example where a child has been very unwell. As Val explains, the severity of Catherine's condition 'dawned on us very slowly'. Catherine had intrauterine growth retardation but appeared to be otherwise well. However, she developed septicaemia during the neo-natal period, and was not well enough to be discharged home until she was two months old. She then developed bronchiolitis and was again very unwell. With this, having gastro-oesophageal reflux, and subsequent chest infections, she spent most of her first year in hospital. As a result, Val explains that a lot of the things that might have alerted her to Catherine having a serious or long-term problem were attributed, by herself, the nurses and Portage workers to her spending most of her first year in hospital. 'People might say "Why couldn't she see? She's got Thomas [Catherine's older brother]?" But Thomas' first year was so different. You just couldn't compare them.' After having a gastrostomy and fundoplication for severe gastro-oesophageal reflux, Catherine was 'well, for the first time in her life'. However, she still failed to develop. 'That was when I realised that she must have severe brain damage and I wanted to know.' While Val accepts that some of the delay in her awareness of the extent of Catherine's problems was 'that I didn't want to know', the confounding factors of her neo-natal illness, respiratory problems, and gastro-oesophageal reflux overshadowed the extent of her long-term problems.

In other cases, it is difficult for families to fully appreciate the enormity of what they are told about their child's condition. Judy was told that Simon would have long-term problems very early on in his life; however, she explains, 'I was completely in shock and couldn't take it in'. Judy describes how, despite what she was told, the reality of the extent of Simon's disabilities was something that she realised very gradually: 'It really hit me when he was about two, when he still didn't walk. His father had bought him a baby walker before he was born, and at 12 months he hadn't used it, and by 18 months he still hadn't used it, and it sat in the corner of the flat, like a bad omen. When he was two, I threw it out.'

Information-giving

Although other events or problems which the child faces may mask the severity of their illness, parents often report that the information which they are given is unclear, incomplete, minimised, or that assumptions are made about what they know, which all delay them realising the extent of their child's problems. Val explains: 'I don't honestly think anyone said to us how ill Catherine was and the effects of this. I had a discussion with the paediatrician when she was still quite little and he said, "I don't think the future looks very rosy for her. I think we're talking about seating systems and mobility equipment." But he never actually said, "She's got brain damage." It was never spelled out.'

Similarly, Debby does not feel that she and Martin were fully informed of the long-term implications of Michael's extreme prematurity. She describes how assumptions seemed to be made about how much information they had and their interpretation of what this meant. They were aware of the issues which Michael faced when withdrawal of treatment was discussed, and understood that his survival was in question. However, the range, magnitude, and long-term implications of his problems were things which they discovered slowly, and often by chance. Although Michael's patent ductus arteriosus (PDA) was mentioned when withdrawal of treatment was discussed, thereafter cardiac problems were not alluded to. Debby discovered that Michael also had an atrial septal defect and pulmonary stenosis when a medical student came to see him on the special care baby unit (SCBU) and asked if she could listen to his heart murmur. The next day Debby and Martin received an appointment for a heart clinic at one of the London hospitals. Until that time, they had assumed, because nothing else had been mentioned to them, that the PDA had closed, and there was no further problem. Debby and Martin were also aware that the assisted ventilation which Michael had required as a neonate had damaged his lungs and that he had residual lung damage. However, it was while they were on the paediatric intensive care unit (PICU), when Michael was less than a year old, that they learnt how badly his lungs had been damaged. Debby explains: 'I am not sure I realised or understood the level of damage done to Michael's lungs until the PICU, with doctors talking of both lower lobes extensively damaged and Michael functioning at 50 per cent lung capacity.' Eventually, after a computerised tomography (CT) scan of his lungs when Michael was four the respiratory consultant explained that he had extensive scarring, limited lung capacity, and that it could be 8–15 years before the scarring reduced to a minimum, and then only if Michael remained free of infections which might cause further damage.

Debby and Martin were also aware of the intraventricular haemorrhages and associated ventricular enlargement that Michael had as a neonate. However, because these were not discussed again, Debby 'thought that they were like a bruise, and after the initial injury, they would get better'. This view was compounded by the fact that 'no one said otherwise, and no one mentioned them again'. However, the day before Michael was leaving the neo-natal intensive care unit (NICU) Debby noticed another baby having a head scan. This prompted her to ask about Michael's bleeds, to confirm that he had fully recovered from them. The reply was, 'No, we don't know if he'll ever walk.' The diagnosis of retinopathy of prematurity (ROP) also came to Debby's attention by chance. She recalls what took place during the handover from the NICU nurse to the SCBU nurse: 'The nurse whom had brought Michael from the NICU was going through his conditions with the nurse in SCBU. Grade 3 retinopathy of prematurity was mentioned. This had never been mentioned to us' (Barrett 2007).

There is also some evidence of assumptions being made that parents will deduce what is wrong with their child or what this means. Mr and Mrs Hethrington had not been told that Lucy was likely to develop seizures. Mr Hethrington recalls: 'She was walking on beach and she went slightly blue and we thought she was cold. But if we'd been told she may start having fits and this is what they may look like, then we would have known.' Mrs Hethrington also recalls the hospital staff being surprised that Lucy was not already receiving anticonvulsants when she was admitted there: 'At the hospital they said: "How come she's not on any [anticonvulsant] medication?"' This left the family feeling 'as if we'd missed something. I felt stupid' although there was no reason for them to know that Lucy might have seizures or what they would look like.

Support During Diagnosis

Receiving the news that your child has a severe and ongoing problem can be, as Rosemary describes, 'heartbreaking'. As well as the information imparted at the time of diagnosis, the manner in which it is conveyed, and the support offered at this time are very important. However, not all families recall being spoken to in a caring or supportive manner. Rosemary describes how she and Colin were made aware of Christian's problems: 'As the neurologist was examining Christian, he suddenly broke off what he was doing, looked up at us, and said "You do realise that this child has got gross mental disability and he's never going to be able to walk or talk." We hadn't got a clue. We just looked at each other and we couldn't speak, I remember quite clearly, we went outside, into the brilliant sunshine and stood on the pavement, Christian in his pushchair. We put our arms around each other, both trying to hold the other one up, and just sobbed and sobbed. We didn't know, we hadn't had a child before. We did not have a clue about "child development" or "milestones". We didn't know.' Cheryl and Steve also describe how they 'met a consultant who used words that no parent should ever have to hear. He had met Hannah once, it was the first time he met her, she was three months old, and he said, "Grieve for the child you thought you had. She won't walk, she probably won't talk, and if she does it'll be a bonus. Oh, and any other kids you have they'll probably be the same."' In Niamh's case, the diagnosis of cerebral palsy was communicated to Rachel by letter rather than in person as she recalls: 'The orthopaedic consultant didn't actually tell me at the time of Niamh's appointment. I don't know what happened but I received the clinic letter and on it was the diagnosis. I was gutted, because I didn't want that diagnosis and it had come in a letter' (Dickinson 2007).

The manner in which the diagnosis is conveyed, the information which accompanies this, and explanation of what the diagnosis means are important for families. Even when there is uncertainty over the precise diagnosis, or likely disease trajectory, families report valuing being given open and honest information. Helen describes the consultant who cared for David in London and continues to provide input is someone for whom she has the greatest respect and trust: 'I value the ones who are honest. At [London Hospital] we saw them and they said this is what is wrong with David, and it is very rare, but we will tell you what we know, and we will go with what we know. They were always very upfront. Some doctors don't feel they can say they don't know, because they feel they should know, but we don't expect them to, with something as rare as this. We do value honesty.'

However, many families have not had positive experiences in relation to being given information. Sharon explains how Zoë was eventually diagnosed as having cerebral palsy: 'He [the paediatrician] basically said, "Yes, she's got cerebral palsy. Bye-bye see you in six months' time." That was it.' Sharon and her husband had very little knowledge of cerebral palsy at the time when Zoë was diagnosed, and 'the only pictures we'd seen of cerebral palsy were the Scope pictures, which are for fundraising. Luckily we'd got a very very good physio who gave me some books.'

Having a Diagnosis

Despite the sadness associated with a child being diagnosed as having a long-term problem, having a diagnosis can have positive aspects. One advantage can be that the problem is identified and, as Mr and Mrs Hethrington explain, 'in some ways it was good to have a name' and something concrete about which they could seek information. Once a diagnosis is made, more specific support can sometimes also be forthcoming. For example, once Michael was diagnosed as having austistic spectrum disorder the autism team became involved with him, and he was allocated someone to work one to one with him for one afternoon a week. Debby and Michael also started attending a support group for children with autism.

Having a diagnosis or clarity over the extent of a problem may also enable families to have reasonable or realistic expectations for their child. Val describes how she changed once she knew the extent of Catherine's brain injury: 'Now, I know, I understand, I don't spend hours trying to teach her stuff she can't learn, I haven't got unreasonable expectations. The brain scan was the thing that finally made me be more realistic about her.' Diagnosis may also help families to prepare better for the future, and to ensure that the care they give is to their child's advantage in the long term. For example, Cheryl and Steve explain, 'we know a lot of girls get scoliosis, so we can be really careful with positioning to guard against that'.

Diagnosis may also be important in making families feel believed and respected. Mrs Hethrington describes how hearing the plastic surgeon's recognition of Lucy's craniostenosis, 'was just a relief, I didn't know what he was going to say, but he didn't say "go out and get a job."' It was the acknowledgement that a problem existed and that Lucy's need would be acted upon, not the diagnosis itself, that was the relief.

The overall picture of diagnosis is therefore one of devastation mixed with relief. As Debby recalls, when Michael was diagnosed as having autistic spectrum disorder: 'I was devastated. Relieved, but devastated. I still don't know how I felt after the diagnosis, I guess a mixture of sadness and relief. The sadness comes in that we kissed ever having "normal" goodbye that day, and once again I'm left grieving for the baby/child I never had. The relief comes in knowing that it wasn't me, and my relationship with Michael that was causing his problems; at last we had an answer and the hope was that this would then open the doors to the help and support that we were so desperate for' (Barrett 2007).

In other respects, however, a label makes no difference to the everyday reality of the child's needs, because, as Mr Hethrington explains, Lucy has the needs she has regardless of the label. A geneticist has recently told the family that Lucy does not have a typical genetic picture of Rett syndrome; however, as Mr Hethrington comments, 'that doesn't make any difference to how she is, she needs the same treatment and care whatever you call it'. In addition, Steve and Cheryl emphasise the importance of still seeing each child as an individual, regardless of their diagnosis: 'We know other girls with Rett syndrome, even the same variant, and Hannah isn't the same. Even though you have a diagnosis, you can't generalise.'

Prognosis

As well as diagnosis, many families feel that being given an indication of their child's likely prognosis is very valuable. Val describes how important information on Catherine's likely prognosis was for her and for her family: 'We [Val and her husband] were talking about the future, and we realised that we had very different attitudes on Catherine's prognosis, because I was saying that as we don't know how long we've got her every day is precious, and Tony was saying: "She's as strong as an ox she's going to outlive us both." We ended up getting very upset because I have always felt she's so vulnerable she could deteriorate at any point. We had a clinic appointment coming up, so we asked the paediatrician, "How long is she going to live?" He said, "Well actually if you'd asked me a few years ago I'd have said her prognosis was less good, but since she's had the gastrostomy and fundoplication she's been well, and her prognosis has got better and I think she'll probably get through school and reach early adulthood."' Val was surprised by his response, given Catherine's vulnerability. 'He said something along the lines of that as caring parents you pick up on things and they'll get treated and sorted out, and I really think you need to think about where she's going to go later on.' Val found his approach very helpful. 'He was saying that at some point you need to have a life of your own, and it might be worth thinking about what her options are when she finishes school, because she'll be with you 24/7. I still feel she is very vulnerable, but I think it was good to make us look at things that way, and I think yes, when Thomas is 18 he's going to leave home, he won't want to live with his parents, so why should she? I suppose it made me think of it from her point of view.'

Despite the importance of knowing the long-term implications and likely outcomes of a child's condition, the information available to medical staff may be incomplete, or new knowledge may emerge which contradicts previous advice. Although associated with risks to future children, rather than Zak or Sophia's prognosis, the information which Cheryl recalls receiving about the recurrence of congenital central hypoventilation syndrome (CCHS) illustrates this point: 'I asked everyone about the chances of having another child with it, and was told there was no chance of it happening again. I was told, "No chance, there's not been anyone in the world that has happened to." And so I had Sophia and she has it worse than Zak. I had been told it was a one in a million chance. I was the first person in the world that this happened to.' Nevertheless, while acknowledging the many unknowns in the world of the child with complex and continuing health needs, Debby explains that as much information as possible is vital for families: 'What we wanted, and didn't get, was for someone to take the time to sit with us, and explain the ins and outs of everything, the positive and the negative, the chances of having a child with long-term issues. What the future could hold for our family. I realise doctors don't have crystal balls and that no one can predict how things will turn out, but the odds would have been good, at least that would have enabled us to make choices, and be prepared for the future. As much as I love my son, one of the main difficulties has always been the uncertainty, the not knowing, the wait and see game we've played. I deal with things far better if I know what I'm dealing with. If I have all the cards laid out in front of me then it is easier to handle. I cannot cope with surprises round every corner' (Barrett 2007).

It is also vital that the information which families are given on prognosis is as up-to-date and accurate as possible. Helen recalls what happened at their local hospital: 'They told us that by the time he went to school David would be fine, he'd have grown out of it [CCHS]. So we went down to London [to discuss David's diagnosis] thinking that and they said, "Well, no, actually, he's got this for life."' Debby and Martin were also given false hopes of how fully Michael would recover from his early start to life. 'We were told very clearly that Michael would have caught up by the time he was two. We clung to this, it was a light at the end of a very long tunnel, what we didn't realise at the time was that light was attached to a train. We have been hit so many times by that train, because information we have been given was wrong' (Barrett 2007). 'Two was when it was all going to be OK. You cling to that light at the end of the tunnel. That magic second birthday when everything will be OK. Then two comes, and three, and four, and you think, "It's not going to happen."'

Summary

Although a child being diagnosed as having a certain condition should not detract from them being seen as an individual and as part of the family, having a diagnosis or clarity over the extent of a child's problems has benefits. These can include clarity over what the problem is, more specific information, and the potential for support becoming available.

However, for many children and their families, obtaining a diagnosis is not a simple or clear-cut process. This may be because their condition is rare or an unusual variant of a condition, or because it does not precisely match any known condition. It can also sometimes be that diagnosis is delayed because medical staff do not fully appreciate the benefit of families knowing the extent of their child's condition or because professionals do not take into account the information which families give them or appreciate the intuitive knowledge that parents have of their child.

The way in which diagnostic processes are handled is very important for children and their families, including the manner in which they are spoken to and the quality of the supporting information that they are given. As well as diagnosis, information on their child's likely prognosis is very important for them and their families. While there will almost always be some degree of uncertainty about their likely prognosis, children and their families having as much accurate information as possible is vital to assist them when planning and making decisions about their lives.

Chapter 7

Support

As described in Chapter 3, parents whose children have complex and continuing health needs carry a significant physical, organisational and emotional workload for 24 hours a day. For this reason, support or assistance in providing the care that their child needs can be extremely beneficial for them, and in many cases is essential to enable their child to live at home. This support can include advice, information, emotional support, or the provision of practical assistance. The type and duration of practical help may vary from short slots of assistance, for example as Debby describes, 'someone to come in and help by looking after Michael to enable me to do the everyday things like play with his siblings, give them some time and attention, and do some basic housework' (Barrett 2007), through to 24-hour assistance with the child's care. Some families also have a facility for short-break or respite care.

The quality of the support which families receive is extremely important; however, it is also very variable. Cheryl and Steve explain that the borough where they now live generally provides a high standard of the type of support which they need. However, one of the reasons for them moving to the area was because the support available in their previous borough was very poor. Other families have reported that support is difficult to access, inadequate, or unreliable, and that the process of trying to obtain assistance is a significant stressor for them. Debby recalls how she has felt when trying to access support: 'I'm not sure I will ever really be able to describe adequately the time I have spent in tears, the sense of isolation, the frustration, the rejection, and the anger'. In addition to the difficulty which some families experience in obtaining support, because this may be the responsibility of a variety of services, parents often have to add co-ordinating the support that their child needs to the other demands on their time.

This chapter describes some of the support that families have experienced and the factors which appear to influence the quality of its provision.

Information and Advice

Parents often need information and advice about specific practical, medical, or technical issues related to their child's care. Cheryl and Steve describe how their current borough provides a comprehensive range of such support, 'a specialist health visitor, physiotherapist, occupational therapist, everything'. In addition, very soon after they moved to their new home the epilepsy nurse visited them and gave them information, including books and DVDs, and 'was fantastic, let us talk, and ask questions. She couldn't answer all the questions, but it was good to just have someone to talk to, and fire off questions to.' However, families do not always receive this level or quality of support, even in relation to the basic practicalities of care. Mrs Hethrington explains, 'nobody has shown me how to change nappies for a 13-year-old, or dress a 13-year-old'. As well as meaning that parents may unnecessarily struggle with practical tasks, Val describes how a lack of information and advice on certain elements of care can constitute a risk to the child's well-being. Catherine had a gastrojejunostomy tube inserted 'on the understanding that we were going to have support in the community, and we've had very little. I don't think the tube is working, and a part of that may be how we are managing it, and so I think that the lack of support has made a difference to the success of the tube.' From the planning stage of Catherine's elective admission for gastrojejunal tube placement, Val requested support and teaching about the use and care of the tube, 'and it was agreed that we would have support. The extra support I knew we would need.' Val was given some advice regarding the tube before leaving hospital, but formal training was to be arranged locally. Val describes how 'Catherine's been home for a month now and we've not had any training.' Although training is now being organised, this has to be done via the trust training department. Although Val acknowledges 'I do understand that, because it has to be right and everyone has to be told the right things and meet standards', getting advice on how the tube should be managed has, in the interim, been hugely problematic with some confusion over what is and is not safe practice.

This lack of information contrasts with the training that staff can expect to receive. As Mrs Hethrington describes, 'people who work in care homes get shown how to do it [change and dress people]. They get training and they are paid, but I got no training at all.' Colin and Rosemary are not only unable to access training themselves, but are expected to provide staff with training about almost all the aspects of Hollie and Christian's care. However, as Rosemary comments: 'Who's to say that what I'm teaching them is the correct or up-to-date method? But I am not allowed to access any of the training. Not even the mandatory training.'

Having Staff in Your Home

Although providing support for families is vital, it often means that they have staff working in or visiting their home on a regular basis. Even when this involves occasional visitors giving advice rather than many hours of practical support it can be intrusive. Sharon recalls how, after Zoë was diagnosed as having cerebral palsy she, 'had a steady stream of visitors. It wasn't really fair on my other daughter and I couldn't go anywhere. I had to make sure I was always back in time for the next one.' At the other end of the spectrum, Rosemary and Colin have a visitor in their home for 24 hours a day to provide Hollie's support. Rosemary explains that this involves three shift changes each day, and two staff per shift change, so that the family have at least six staff in their house each day, for seven days a week.

Although the remit of support staff is to decrease parents' workload, their presence can be exhausting, on top of an already demanding schedule. Jo describes how the effort of socialising with staff can take time and energy which she can ill afford: 'What I find hard sometimes is when they want to have a chat. People will come and you have to chit-chat and get filled in on other people's news and that can sometimes be quite draining, because it happens in the morning and the evening and it can go on for half an hour.' There can also be a degree of discomfort for parents over their role when they have assistance with childcare at home. Jo describes how when she has assistance during the day, for example during Mitchell's school holidays, she can feel guilty at taking time for herself, to do her work, while someone else looks after Mitchell: 'I feel really uncomfortable about going and doing my studying, I kind of wander back and forwards between the lounge and my study, feeling like I'm not sure what I should be doing.'

Having professional visitors in the house also means that the family's life is no longer private. As Jo describes, 'it is like being in a goldfish bowl: everything can be watched'. The degree to which this is a problem depends to a great extent on the amount of time that staff are in the home, on individual staff, and the family's preferences. Helen describes how she differs from some mothers who 'are really good friends with the staff and form friendships with them, but we don't, we tend to keep our distance from them'. For Helen, this is very important; for her, the ideal staff are those who are interested in providing the right care for David, but do not seek to become involved with the family. 'We have got two who are like chalk and cheese, one who will come in and say "Hello, how are you? How's David? Any changes? Fine." And then she goes and gets on with it. We've got another one who comes in and says things like "You look nice, have you been out?" and if I say yes, she says "Oh, anywhere nice?" She said to David "Oh, I like your pyjamas, where did you get them from? I want to get some for my son." Or she'll say, "You've got a new car?" or "I can smell paint are you decorating?"' This level of interest is irrelevant to David's care, and it feels like an intrusion on the family's privacy.

Some families describe the measures that they have taken to manage the intrusion of having staff in their homes. Judy, who has 24-hour assistance from care staff, explains, 'we're very lucky in that the carer has a separate little annexe because if she lived in the house it would be more difficult'. Helen also describes how they have designed their home to minimise the intrusion which staff, of necessity, create. This includes installing an intercom to her and John's room so that staff can contact them this way rather than coming to their room at night; David's room being situated so that staff do not have to walk through the house to get to it; a separate sitting room beside David's room so that he has his privacy and the staff have a sitting room away from the family. Helen explains: 'Before we moved they had to come through the house to his room and that was quite difficult. You felt as if you had got to have the house tidy all the time. When we moved we moved with it in mind that we wanted this set-up, and it has worked.'

One challenge for service providers and families can be achieving the balance between providing adequate support without creating too great an intrusion on the family. In addition, how families will be enabled to bond with, feel ownership of, and develop expertise in their child's care while also being supported must be considered. Helen explains how, despite the apparent benefits of having 24-hour support, complete reliance on support staff can become problematic because, 'a nurse whose job it is to look after your child on a one-to-one basis is automatically going to do everything for that child, and this means that parents do not get the experience of the nursing side of their child's care'. Helen adds that this type of situation can mean that if support staff become unavailable, for example due to sickness, the child may have to be admitted to hospital until the staff become available again.

In addition to the physical intrusion, having staff working in their home means that the family can become involved in employment and disciplinary matters, which can be very stressful. Alison recalls: 'We've got some fantastic care staff, some really really good staff who are like family but we've also had some nightmares. We've had people fall asleep on duty and sleep through alarms, and I've had to report that. You feel awful because you're having to be like a boss, but you just want to be a Mum.' Another issue, especially when carers have a high level of input, can be maintaining the boundaries between being a friend and an employer or work colleague. Judy explains, 'this [current] carer is very close to my age and we get on very well and it's difficult to keep the employer not friend boundaries'.

Short-break Services

In addition to day-to-day support, respite or short-break facilities are vital for families. However, such facilities are often scarce or difficult to access. Cheryl has no short-break care for Zak and Sophia. She describes how she has 'tried and tried until I am blue in the face, but there's nothing'. It took Debby and Martin four years to obtain any daytime care for Michael. They can now have up to 12 days per year, but still have no overnight care. During the four years it took for respite care to materialise, Michael started school, making daytime respite care less vital for the family. However, as Debby and Martin explain, they make sure that they use this facility 'or else it will go, and when we do need it, it won't be there'. This concern illustrates that many families are aware of the pressure on existing support mechanisms. For example, Catherine's family has been assessed as needing one night a week and one weekend in six short-break care, which is provided at the respite care unit at the local hospital. They can also access up to 12 nights a year care at the local children's hospice. However, staff shortages mean that their regular nights at the hospital unit are not 100 per cent reliable and the 12 nights a year at the hospice are becoming more difficult to arrange as the demands on their resources increase. Val explains: 'When Catherine first came out of hospital, we had our regular one night a week respite cancelled due to staff sickness and failure to train other staff in the use of the [gastrojejunostomy] tube.' Although this provision has now resumed, Catherine's weekend respite care was only restarted several weeks after her surgery because of staff sickness. Val recalls: 'We were supposed to have our first weekend of respite for eight months after Catherine came home from hospital and they just cancelled it. Fortunately, we hadn't booked anything but only because I hadn't got around to booking anything. I understand that they are short-staffed but they can never understand the effect on our family of cancelled respite.'

As well as a lack of respite care facilities, some service providers do not appear to appreciate the impact of having a child with complex and continuing health needs and the necessity of short-break care. Alison has only recently been able to access any short-break care for Peter because, 'initially, they said I didn't need respite. They thought because I have night care I don't need respite. Social services didn't see it as a need. But when you've got a child who's ventilated, like Peter, you need two trained carers on the premises. So even though I've got night care, I can't leave him, I have to be here 24/7. They don't understand that.'

Quality of Support

As well as the amount, the quality of the support which is provided is very important for children and their families. Staff who provide support need to be competent, but providing support that sees the child as a person and part of the family, with needs outside their healthcare is also vital. In some cases, staff are clearly aware of this. Steve and Cheryl report that their occupational therapist has provided a portable bath for Hannah to use at the gym which the family uses, because 'she said her job is to help Hannah in all settings, not just at home'. However, in other instances parents do not feel that staff see the importance of meeting their child's needs as a person. Rosemary estimates that of the nine staff who regularly work with Hollie, 'I would say there are two who appreciate that Hollie is a person, and Hollie has a life outside of medical procedures. The others seem to see themselves as being there to do nursing tasks and they don't think that Hollie might want to do something, to play, to be educated. She might want to read a book, and not be read to but join in the reading so that she can practise her reading abilities. She is not being allowed to direct her own life. To direct what she wants to do each day. It's more about tracheostomy care, giving nebulisers, drugs, feeds, doing suction, and an unbelievable obsession regarding the completion of nursing notes. Doing tasks. Not about Hollie.'

The quality of support is also affected by the extent to which staff respect families and their knowledge, views, preferences and priorities, and thus how far parents can really trust staff to care for their child. Rosemary describes how Hollie requires careful postural care to treat her scoliosis, but that few staff are fully committed to providing this. She explains how, in order to be effective, 'it's got to be consistent and not done to appease the mother and we'll do it when we think she's looking and then turn her over on her side in the most horrendous postural position possible because she's not watching'.

As well as individual staff, organisational issues have a major impact on the quality of the support which families receive. There was a general feeling among families that the support which they need is often unavailable because there does not appear to be the capacity for this within the services. Alison's experience has led her to believe that the National Health Service has done very little forward thinking in relation to the increasing number of children who will have continuing care needs: 'They haven't thought about the effect on the community services. It's going to be more common. These children are going to survive. That needs to be looked at as a matter of urgency.' Debby also explains that, 'support services are not set up to deal with the long-term issues thrown up by the number of extremely premature infants' (Barrett 2007).

One specific problem in the provision of support is staff availability. Rosemary explains: 'Finding staff is a difficult process, especially in view of complex healthcare needs. When one looks at the job description, the qualifications and training a person would need to look after Christian, they would have to be near nursing standards. Hollie, having a tracheostomy, is an even more difficult case to assess.' Even when staff can be found, Cheryl explains that there is a problem with retaining staff: 'We have had two carers who have been with us from before Sophia was born, but apart from those two we've never really been able to keep staff. They stay 18 months or two years and they get to know them, and then you have to start all over again, getting to know them and training them. You just get used to somebody and they go.'

In some cases, poor organisation or administration of services contributes to families not receiving assistance. Debby recalls that it took four months of lost files and unreturned telephone calls to the Social Services Department before Michael was assessed for shared care. He was then on a waiting list for four years. After three years the family was offered a shared carer, but the person who was allocated to them was not sufficiently mobile to be able to catch Michael, which, given his problems, was an essential part of her work. This illustrates the importance of assessing the child and family's precise needs and matching the support provided to this. In other instances, too, services may not meet a child or family's needs because organisational processes do not appear to take into account the practicality of arrangements or how far they will actually assist families. For example, Helen recalls: 'One year they were going to have a major cutback on the budget and have the staff coming in at 11pm and going at 6am. That would mean that by the time they come in at 11, and you hand over it's a quarter past eleven, I then go and have my bath, and I've got to be up again at five. How little sleep are you supposed to manage on?'

Many families also report that service providers do not appear to appreciate the magnitude of having a child with complex and continuing health needs. Helen explains how some providers view the support which families receive as a luxury, not a necessity: 'They conveyed "You're lucky you're getting the support every night." But we're not lucky; we need it.' Cheryl also describes how 'the carers do understand how it is, the effect on your life and their lives. Those in control don't appreciate how hard it is. The carers say: "How the hell do you do this?" The people who are doing it appreciate it, but those in charge are not actually coming and doing it themselves.' In addition, the way in which services are prioritised may disadvantage children with complex and continuing health needs. Val recounts: 'In the community team's eyes Catherine is not ill, she's not a priority; in fact, I was told by the community team: "We are really stretched looking after a terminally ill child." And I thought, "That says it all. She's not ill, it doesn't matter."'

The quality of care or support which children receive may also be affected by the extent to which its organisation enables staff to care for one child consistently, or to match staff to the child and family. Judy describes how, when Simon was younger, she had a carer from the local authority to assist her, but that they could not guarantee that the same person would assist her all the time. As Judy explains, this meant that the support which she received and the care provided for Simon was less than acceptable because 'continuity with a child like Simon is really important. You totally need continuity. The medical side aside, he gets used to someone and with his communication, he needs someone who knows him.'

As well as continuity, the close working relationship between families and support staff makes it important that they can work well together. Ideally this means identifying what relationship the family wants: some families may prefer minimal involvement and a professional but distant relationship, whereas others may prefer more friendship or involvement. In addition, the nature of the child's needs can make developing relationships very lengthy and labour intensive. Jo explains: 'Mitchell's got to develop a whole new relationship. In a way because of his level of disability there's a relationship that is with him and a bit that has to come through me. They need to get on with both of us. It takes ages. We need to work together, there's a process of him establishing his relationship, but me facilitating that, saying this is what's happening. It's tiring. It's emotionally quite draining.' However, in most cases, unless families have a means of employing staff themselves (such as direct payments), it is unusual for them to be involved in the appointment of support staff and Jo comments: 'Managerially, they see numbers: what they don't realise is these are all relationships and every one is different and you have to really work on establishing that. It's not just replacing one person with another.' Jo describes how, when staff are appointed, 'sometimes you can tell right away if they are right for Mitchell, if they're really quiet, he's really quiet: never the twain shall meet. What you need is someone who will talk but also in a way that allows him to get into the relationship. Sort of chatty but calm. There are certain sort of qualities that he seems to gel well with, which, as his Mum, I would be able to identify.' Like all aspects of decision-making regarding support, the important thing is to ascertain what families would prefer in relation to staff appointments, and facilitate this. Helen has always opted to leave staff recruitment to the organisation that provides the staff. This has involved balancing the advantages and disadvantages: 'Part of me doesn't want to get involved in that side of things, but, on the other hand, I feel bit like there are people coming into my house whom I don't know, but we have just accepted that we have the staff they send.'

As well as the quality of day-to-day support, many parents describe the importance, but comparative paucity, of back-up plans. Cheryl explains that if the staff who usually provide Zak and Sophia's night care are not available at short notice (for example, owing to sick leave) the only back-up she has is her mother, 'but she can't do the ventilation side of it. Especially with Sophia [whose condition is worse and whose sleep pattern is less predictable than Zak's].' Where parents have more than one child, back-up plans need to take this, as well as the potential for staff sickness, into account. Cheryl recalls a time when Zak became acutely unwell and had to be admitted to hospital. Cheryl's only assistance during Zak's admission and the days and evenings while he was in hospital was her mother. As Cheryl's mother is not confident to institute Sophia's assisted ventilation, on the evening when Zak was being admitted she had to keep Sophia awake until half-past nine, when the carers arrive. This was a struggle and Cheryl had to telephone constantly to ensure that everything was all right while she was managing Zak's admission. Cheryl explains that this situation illustrates that, 'actually it doesn't take much to tip things over. There is no back-up.'

Staff Training

To provide support for families, staff need to be competent in all aspects of the child's care. One issue that can affect the quality of the support offered therefore is the quality of staff training. However, organising and facilitating this can be problematic. The support that Hollie and Christian receive comes predominantly from staff who are employed by an agency, which creates a problem for training. Rosemary explains, 'strictly speaking the primary care trust should do it, but they will not train agency staff'.

Second, Rosemary explains that most agencies do not pay their staff to attend training. Staff have to attend mandatory training, regardless of whether or not they are paid, because they cannot work without it. However, any non-mandatory training is at their discretion, and therefore if they are not paid to attend, many will not do so. Thus, 'even if the PCT [primary care trust] did provide training, agency staff will not go to the training because they're not going to be paid for it. So you're at stalemate.' An example of this problem is training for one very vital aspect of Hollie and Christian's care: postural care. This does not form a part of mandatory training, and is therefore not provided by the agency. However, Rosemary organised a study day on postural care and positioning for the staff, which the facilitator agreed to put on at no cost to participants (the usual cost would be approximately £100 per person). None of the staff from the agency attended because they were not paid to do so. Similarly, no training can be arranged on tracheostomy care, suctioning, gastrostomy feeding, administration of rectal diazepam and buccal midazolam, physiotherapy, and other medical and technical procedures. This situation leads Rosemary to ask, 'where does the clinical governance lie? Would it be with myself, or with the care agency, or perhaps the PCT? A medical procedure carried out incorrectly, such as suctioning a tracheostomy, could lead to death.' In addition, Rosemary explains that training related to some aspects of nursing care as well as medical or technical procedures should be mandatory, for example communication and 'person-centred awareness is essential'.

Establishing Support

Establishing the support which parents need in order to enable their child to be cared for at home can be very difficult. As described in Chapter 3 this can significantly delay a child's initial discharge from hospital. For example, Helen recalls how David's discharge from the local hospital was a very lengthy and problematic process, principally because of the time which it took to organise the necessary support services and to train staff. 'That was a very, very difficult time. It was a case of they had never had a child like this in this area, and had never had to set up this kind of thing and we kept being told we had to be patient.' Eventually, 'David came home, but only after the consultant whose care he was under in London pushing the local health authority [as it then was] and encouraging us to push them. In the end the consultant threatened to go to the papers saying that this child is taking up an acute bed, this is costing so much, and he should be at home. We didn't have to go to the papers, but I think we would have done if we had to. It was a real nightmare, but it's something we went through and eventually did get him home.'

Changes in a child's age can also mean that support services have to be reviewed and reorganised, creating an element of uncertainty for them and their families. For example, David's night support is currently provided by staff from the children's hospice. However, once he is transferred to adult services this will cease and the most likely outcome is that the primary care trust will contract his support to an agency.

When a child's clinical state changes it can mean that home care will be re-funded and re-organised again, becoming problematic and having to be renegotiated. For Hollie, needing an emergency tracheostomy when she was close to transition to adult services meant that she spent six months in hospital because of debates about the funding and practicalities of her care at home both because of her changed needs and her transition to adult services. Eventually, after the family explored every possible avenue it was agreed that Hollie would be provided with full-time nursing cover at home, but, as Rosemary explains this was only 'because we got uppity about "Valuing People" and "Care in the Community" and the child's right to be within their own home. We went really quite high and threatened legal action. Eventually, the integrated services commissioner for learning disabilities for adults, even though Hollie was still in paediatrics, agreed that, just to get her out of hospital and to stop all the legalities we were threatening, learning disabilities would pay to provide nursing care at home. But we still haven't got a contract saying that this is definitely what will happen. We are just literally limping along, still with no agreement that this is what has been assessed as being needed. We fear on a daily basis, that this care will stop.'

Other Support

In many cases, support for parents comes primarily from their family and friends. This may be their choice, or because of a lack of other options. Some families do not want a great deal of day-to-day practical support as

Cheryl explains: 'We probably could have more [support] but we don't really want strangers coming into our house. I don't even want someone coming into my house to do my ironing. I am the sort of person that if I had a cleaner I would have to clean first.' Steve explains that they may need assistance at a later date 'when Hannah's older, and heavier' but at the moment they prefer to care for Hannah with support from family and friends. Although some families choose to manage without a great deal of assistance, because they cope a family can sometimes become low priority for assistance. Val recalls how a paediatrician once apologised to her for not offering the family a great deal of support but explained, 'you always seem to cope so well'. Similar sentiments have been expressed by the community nursing team. Val questions how these people know that they are coping, or how they define coping, 'People say, "I am amazed how you cope," and I think, "Well how do you know I'm coping?"'

However, accepting help with direct care for their child from family and friends is not what every family wants or sees as appropriate, and should not be an expectation. For example, Helen explains, 'I never felt comfortable asking family or friends to look after David. I think the main thing was the fits he was having because they were life-threatening. I had a friend who did offer to train up to look after him, but I said no because if anything happened and she didn't deal with that, how would she feel, how would I feel, how would I feel towards her? If it was a nurse, I could hate her, and blame her, she was nobody to me, but it would be more difficult with a friend. So I never ever left him with family or friends.'

In many cases parents gain their most important social and emotional support from other parents whose children have complex and continuing health needs. Val recounts how the support group Proactive Parents has, 'really helped me, enabled me to meet other parents who are struggling to bring up disabled children. We all support each other.' Often, peer support groups are the only place where parents feel understood. Evelyn recalls: 'I don't think I had anyone who truly understood what was wrong with Siobhan. That's why I got into the internet [support groups] eventually, [in the last year or so] because there I met people who just got it.' Other parents also report that the internet can be an invaluable source of support as Judy explains: 'I think you really really need that because a lot of times there aren't really many people in your area, or you don't want to meet up with people in your area.'

Summary

Although the provision of appropriate support to enable children with complex and continuing health needs to live at home with their families is essential, the provision for this and its quality is very variable.

The quality, as well as the amount, of support that families receive is important and is affected by staff seeing the child as a person and part of a family, and respecting families' decisions about their child's care. In addition, organisational and administrative issues, funding arrangements, staff being well matched to the child and family, and consistency of care being ensured affects the quality of the support which families receive. Families also need access to reliable short-break care and planned support to include back-up options.

Although support is vital for families, having staff in their home environment can be difficult for families as Helen describes: 'David and his medical condition are the least of our problems, it is the support that is the problem, and people don't see that. We couldn't have coped without it, but, on the other hand, I would say that it is the thing that gives me the most stress. Having to have staff in our house. People say: "Aren't you lucky, you have a nurse in your home every night. Aren't you lucky you get all this support?" but I think, "No." Yes, it does mean that David has been able to live at home, but having to have the staff has given us more stress than David's medical condition has.'

Chapter 8

Healthcare

Children who have complex and continuing health needs, and their families, often have numerous dealings with healthcare professionals. Specific situations related to this, for example, diagnosis and the provision of support, have been discussed earlier. Some more general points that families have made, which merit consideration for individual practitioners and health service organisations, are discussed here.

Respect

A major issue in the quality of the relationship between healthcare staff and families is whether parents feel that they and their children are respected.

Respect for Expert Knowledge

One important aspect of respect is whether staff respect the expert knowledge that parents have about their child. In some cases, parents report very effective and respectful partnerships with professionals in their child's care. Debby notes her experience at one hospital: 'I feel like we are a part of the team. It feels like we're talked to and involved in everything that goes on and are respected as parents and partners.' Helen also describes a consultant who works in partnership with the family, with each person contributing on an equal footing to decision-making, 'He will say, when David has sleep studies, what do you think, is it positional, what is it? When David needed a change in his ventilation, and he needed to change ventilator, they gave us a list of ones to try and we did it all at home. You have to have something that works for you, and David was trialling them in his normal environment, not in a strange environment in hospital, where he doesn't sleep well anyway. We had a rep who came out to us, we trialled them and picked out the one that David liked and was best for him.'

However, parents do not always feel that they are afforded this degree of respect, and describe how a lack of effective partnership working with professionals can adversely affect the quality of their child's care. Martin and Debby remember how the staff at one hospital failed to respect and act upon their knowledge of Michael, and this has led to inappropriate interventions being given and appropriate treatment being delayed. Martin explains that when Michael develops respiratory problems the staff, 'insist on giving him nebulisers, as if Michael was asthmatic' despite Martin telling them that while a nebuliser will raise Michael's oxygen saturation level, the effect is transient and does not address the underlying problem. Evelyn also describes how parents not being listened to can delay treatment. 'Siobhan's nose use to run 24 hours a day. When she was two she had her tonsils and adenoids out, and her nose stopped running. Then later her nose started running again and I went to the doctor, and they kept giving me nose drops. I kept saying: "Her adenoids have grown back" but no one would listen to me. Eventually the paediatrician sent me to the ENT doctor and I said, "her adenoids have grown back" and he said, "it's highly unlikely". Eventually he agreed to have a look. He came back to me, and he never apologised, but he said not only had her adenoids grown back, they were extremely large again. It took me a year to get someone to listen to me. I could see the doctor basically dismissing me as some mad woman: how could she possibly know?'

Respect for parents' knowledge of their child as well as their child's condition is important in developing good relationships and ensuring that appropriate treatment is given. Steve describes attending a hearing test with Hannah: when Hannah's hearing was being tested Steve could identify when she heard sounds because she stopped sucking her dummy. However, she did not turn to indicate her response and the audiologist did not appear to take note of his observations, resulting in Hannah's hearing being inaccurately assessed. In a similar situation, Chris describes when Mollie has her hearing tested. 'You try saying to them, "She's got cerebral palsy, she can't sit up properly" so they do hearing tests, and because she doesn't move they say she can't hear. OK, she has a hearing problem, we're not being naïve, we know she has a problem, but we are convinced that if they listened to us and to how she responds to certain things they wouldn't assume the diagnosis is that she is profoundly deaf.' Chris emphasises that they do not want Mollie to suffer, but equally they do not want her to have invasive and irreversible surgery such as cochlearl implants unless they are sure it really is the best treatment for her, based on an accurate diagnosis.

Although all the parents commented on the importance of staff respecting their expertise; equally, they do not expect staff to abdicate all responsibility to them as Jo explains. 'There is this emphasis on "Mum knows best" and we do know; we know something's wrong, but we're not in a position to say exactly what it is, and what the intervention should be. I have spoken to some of the nurses, and said that if we come to hospital it's because I am not able to cope at home. So you need to know that I, we as a family, are feeling vulnerable, something is happening that is out of my control, that is making me anxious. I am the expert, yes I am, but I am also looking to you, for us, to combine our expertise. So to leave us, to say, "Oh well, he's 14, she knows what she's doing" isn't always an acknowledgement of the fact that we are seeking help.' Alison also describes how she can tell them what she knows, the scenario, but she expects them then to come back with a solution. 'I know a bit about ventilation, but I don't have a medical degree, so I can tell them that the CO_2 is really high, his oxygen levels are low, I can tell them his secretions are green or whatever, and I give them that information and I expect them to come back and say "Oh, he's got an infection, we'll change the ventilator settings."'

Respect for People

Whether staff see and respect parents and their children as people is also vital to establishing good working relationships. Helen describes how highly she values professionals who, 'when we go and see them, look at the big picture, see how David is, ask about school, his social life, holidays. Others look at David and the ventilator and ask how many alarms we have at night, but they don't see David. They don't want to know about the big picture. That does make a lot of difference. You almost differentiate the doctors who want to know about David and those who aren't interested in anything except what his pressures are and how much oxygen he's having.

David's medical condition does affect his whole life and our lives. So that is quite important to see the whole person and the family.'

Chris also explains the contrast between staff who are very competent and those who are competent and caring. He describes the contrast between two very competent consultants in the NICU. 'One consultant obviously had very good knowledge, but was very clinical. You got the impression that Mollie was just another baby. Then we had another consultant…it was thanks to him, too, that Mollie made quicker progress than she should have. She'd been on a ventilator for 14 weeks, and he made the decision to try her on CPAP [continuous positive airway pressure]. That day he was finishing at about eight o'clock and he stayed until half-past twelve, just for her.' Chris continues, 'Mollie is our little girl. One of the consultants couldn't even remember Mollie's name, and that really annoyed me. They had a week on call each, and she'd been there so long and he said, "How's the baby?" It is a little thing, but the importance is huge. If she was in for a day, fine, but she was there for five months.'

Respect for individuals includes respecting their time. One thing that Cheryl has noticed is, 'when they say they'll try and get back to you today, and they don't'. She continues: 'When I was at work, I know there were a number of times I said that to parents, but when people rang me at work they weren't the most important thing on my to do list, but for me, I am the most important person and if you say you're going to ring me back, don't not ring me back because I may be waiting in for that call. Its all false promises. It's something I've learnt.' Equality and respect is also something that Cheryl has highlighted to her previous employer as being important when meetings are organised. 'We had a meeting with the doctors, nurses, the epilepsy nurse, and the health visitor. They were all there already and all sat down and we walked in, and they all went quiet. They were probably just talking about what they did last night, but it was the most awful feeling. So I have recommended (to my ex-employer) that when people go into meetings, we all go in together, and we all sit down together. And if someone does get there first they leave the door wide open so it's all very informal.' Respect includes respecting all family members and not making assumptions about their involvement in their child's life. For example, Steve finds that despite him organising his work so as to be able to attend almost all of Hannah's appointments, professionals tend to talk to Cheryl, not him. He recalls an occasion when he, Cheryl and Hannah were at an appointment. Hannah was sitting on his lap, however, the doctor said that it was nice to see 'Hannah and her Mum'.

A major problem occurs when professionals appear not to value children because of their needs. For example, Judy describes how 'some people kind of write Simon off. There are some things, medically wise, that we have wanted to try and it's as if, "Well, it's not really worth doing it for Simon."' The family wanted see if a ketogenic diet would improve Simon's epilepsy but Judy explains 'we were fobbed off and fobbed off'. Eventually, Simon commenced a ketogenic diet – with good results. Rosemary also recalls an incident when Christian was seen by a urologist when he was six years old: 'He said, "Ah yes, Christian's testicles haven't descended, but it's not as if he's ever going to have children is it? But if you do feel a lump at any time do come back to me."' In contrast, when a doctor at Great Ormond Street Hospital saw Christian [about having a gastrostomy and fundoplication] and was told what the previous doctor had said, 'He went absolutely ballistic: "What right has that doctor to say that Christian has not got the human right to have children, disabilities or not?" He said not only that, he has a greatly increased risk of testicular cancer. So, the poor child had his testicles done and a fundoplication and a gastrostomy.' Rachel also explains that the nature of a child's needs can be a source of inequality in care provision. 'Niamh's got special needs, but she isn't seen as important because she's got special needs, not a medical problem. I can tell the difference in how she's treated and how the others are treated because she's got a learning disability, not a physical problem. I see how they are all treated and she is treated differently.'

Communication

The manner in which healthcare professionals communicate with families is very important. Chris describes how, even in the worst possible situation, when their son Bailey died, the consultant who was caring for him demonstrated excellent communication and caring skills: 'I cannot fault how he went about it, talking about everything, things like post-mortems, the way he conducted himself in that very very difficult process, I cannot fault him.' However, in other cases, communication can be a source of great dissatisfaction. Rachel recalls attending a multi-disciplinary meeting about Emmy failing to gain weight: 'They ganged up on me, and they were asking me if I fed Emmy. The consultant said, "Are you feeding her?" I said how dare he, that I had been with her when she was dying, and been through all that and you ask me am I feeding her. The nurses were backing him up and saying, "What he means is, is she getting all her feeds?" And I said, "That's not what he said. He said: Are you feeding her? He is 30+ years old, he is quite capable of saying what he means. If he meant was she getting all the feeds, he should have said that." I was just thinking he might say that to another parent who couldn't take it. He should not have said it in that way.'

Some parents also highlight how the effect of thoughtless comments by professionals can last far beyond the encounter, as Evelyn recalls. 'When we were in intensive care, a baby in the next crib had just died. You can imagine what the mood was like. The paediatric cardiologist was very upset and he came over and said to me, "I just want to tell you, don't get your hopes up." I just looked at him and he walked away. You know when you are just so startled you just sit there, and can't say anything. Then I just got up and left, and I cried and cried. And I cried all night. And it has never ever left me. He came over the next day and started to walk over to me and I said, "Don't you even come near me. I don't want to hear you; I don't care what you say, Siobhan is going to be OK. She is going home." But it has never left me. Six years later, I still hear it, and whenever something happens I hear it and I think, "Is that what he meant? Don't get your hopes up that she'll live, or don't get your hopes up that she'll do this or that?" Really, I know he didn't mean any of that. He was having a bad day and some other poor family had been devastated and he took it out on me. But that has never left me.'

Giving Information

As well as the quality of communication, whether parents are given adequate and timely information is important. This includes information on the day-to-day practicalities of their child's care and what they can expect. For example, when Michael was in hospital as a neonate, Debby recalls arriving on the NICU and seeing a blanket over Michael's incubator and the CPAP machine, on which he had relied, gone. 'I thought he'd died while I was on the way over to the hospital. But they said, "Oh no, he's just in oxygen" but my heart was pounding because I thought he'd died. I'd gone back God knows how many weeks to where we were, when he was three weeks old and facing withdrawal of treatment.' In contrast, Debby describes how the intention, manner and back-up arrangements made by staff can make giving information effective and leave the family feeling respected and fully involved even when things go wrong. She describes a time when Michael had been transferred from the local NICU to another hospital for a hernia repair (which, in the event, could not be performed) and an echocardiogram. One of the consultants had done the echocardiogram, but before he could discuss the results with Debby and Martin, Michael was unexpectedly transferred back to the local hospital because the hospital to which he had been transferred had to accept an emergency admission. Debby recalls how, on Michael's arrival back at the local hospital, the nurse escorting him told her, 'Dr X sends his apologies, he did the echo on Michael, and he apologises for not being able to give you the results himself.' The results were given to the family, and in addition, 'when we went back for the second attempt at the hernia repair Dr X came over, introduced himself, and said "I'm Dr X, I am so sorry I couldn't give you the results of the echo myself, but here they are." Wow! My respect for them increased 100 per cent for this.'

In addition to day-to-day events, the overall level of information which parents are given about their child is important because, as Debby explains, 'we have to make decisions about our lives and our children's'. However, parents have reported that the information which they are given is not always complete and in some cases important aspects of it are omitted, possibly because assumptions are made about what other staff have told parents or because of a lack of communication between staff. The result can be that, as Debby explains, 'a lot of important things, we just happened to find out'. This can become not only an issue about communication, but about respect for parents' ownership of their child. As Debby recalls, after discovering a range of important matters about Michael's condition (described earlier in Chapter 6) by chance, 'I cornered the Registrar and said, "Right, start at the top and go down, and tell me everything *you* know about *my* child."'

Another concern may be whether professionals are honest, including being truthful about unknowns or their own limitations. Where families feel that staff are not honest it can taint the relationship with them. Chris and Tracy recall the one event which clouds their impression of the neo-natal unit where Bailey and Mollie were cared for. An incident occurred in which the valve in Mollie's oxygen delivery apparatus was faulty, and for two and a half hours she was without oxygen. Mollie subsequently had to return to the intensive care unit. Tracy says, 'they blamed it on a virus, but we knew it was being without oxygen'. Chris adds, 'I would have preferred it of they had owned up. It was human error. I probably would have said OK. But the culture of litigation, I think, meant that they couldn't own up. I would have accepted that. I could accept that better than covering up.'

Hospitalisation

Many children with complex and continuing health needs spend a considerable amount of time in hospital and this therefore forms an important part of the experience which they and their families have of healthcare.

Most families report that hospital services are so stretched that staff are unable to provide the day-to-day care that their children need, as Debby describes: 'In hospital, a lot of the time the nurses are so busy that they don't have time, so we give Michael all his care. They do medical care, but we do the day-to-day care.' This means that many parents feel unable to leave their children while they are in hospital and, as Val describes, where a child has complex and continuing health needs this can mean being unable to leave the ward even for a few moments: 'Catherine can't speak for herself, she can't even say, "It hurts", so she is totally dependent on you. I can't leave her. I try to get friendly with the other Mums in the bay so that when I go to the loo I can say to them: "If Catherine cries, can you push her buzzer?" So it is totally exhausting.' This is not always the case, as Val clarifies: 'We made a decision when Catherine was tiny and in our local hospital a lot that we would come home to sleep. They all know her really well now and support this. They know her so well I feel able to leave her. Also, it is only ten minutes from home.' This is not, as Val describes above, the case when Catherine is in other hospitals, where she and her family are less well known and where their home is further away.

Parents can also feel that they need to stay with their child because subtle signs of changes in their condition may be missed by staff. Jo reports how her role when Mitchell is in hospital includes 'drawing attention to things when I can see they're changing'. Sometimes parents also feel unable to leave because staff are not familiar with their child's condition. Cheryl describes how the staff at Stoke Hospital frequently deal with children who have congenital central hypoventilation syndrome, and are confident in Zak and Sophia's care. However, the staff at the local children's hospital are less confident and 'when they're in the Children's Hospital the staff convey [to Cheryl] "Don't go home."'

Despite needing to be with their child when they are in hospital, many parents report difficulty in accessing basic requisites such as food and sleep in hospitals. Val explains, 'it is difficult to leave the ward long enough to get a proper meal, so you are stuck with sandwiches'. Evelyn also describes how providing better facilities for parents to sleep would improve the experience of hospitalisation immeasurably: 'They could do away with the chairs [the large chairs beside the child's bed that parents have to use to sleep in]. I know it's hard for space and money but there's nothing worse, when you've got a sick child, than having to sleep in a chair. When you're trying to sleep and you move your legs and the next thing you're sitting bolt upright. You can't sleep. And you've got nurses coming in and out, so you get no sleep, but you've still got to look after your child all day. I remember once when I walked in and I saw that that was where I had to sleep, and I thought, "I just cannot do that chair again."' Evelyn explains how this might seem a small thing, but 'having to cope with no sleep, and looking after a sick child all day, is hard'.

Caring for a sick child in hospital all day is very demanding, but is something which parents have to do, often unaided, with few of the child's familiar activities to distract them, and in a confined environment. Evelyn describes how, on top of having little or no sleep, 'you are with them all day, and you're trying to amuse a toddler on oxygen, and you've got to amuse them all day. They're not able to move because they're on oxygen, and they're not well, but you've got to amuse them all day, and its hard, hard work.'

There is also a suggestion that the stretched service cannot provide for the child and family's basic needs in terms of supplies, and families have to bring into hospital everything that they and their child need. Val recalls Catherine's most recent admission to hospital: 'I don't know how many trips I made from the ward to the car. I have to take her milk, her nappies; at first they provided that but now I have to take it all.' Val also had to bring her own duvet and pillow so that she could stay overnight with Catherine.

When parents stay with their child in hospital they still have to manage the rest of their lives. Mr and Mrs Hethrington describe how, when Lucy is in hospital, as well as one of them staying with her all night and the other staying with her during the day, they also have to do all the usual household chores, such as shopping and laundry (they have to bring Lucy's and their own laundry home). Where parents have more than one child, there is also the consideration of organising the other children's activities. When Catherine is hospitalised, Val's husband has to take Thomas to school and collect him. However, although he is self-employed and able to work fairly flexibly, this can only be managed for a short time, and if Catherine's hospitalisation is prolonged, Val's mother usually comes down to assist. In some cases a child being in hospital can affect their parents' employment and income. For example, on one occasion when Lucy was admitted to hospital, Mr Hethrington had to take time off work and was dismissed because it was his child, not him, that was sick. He became unemployed, but was not eligible for any benefits, because it was Lucy, not him, who was ill. The family spent 12 weeks without income of any kind.

The experience of being in hospital with one's child can be very isolating for parents, and families may be restricted in supporting one another by distance or hospital regulations. Catherine's most recent admission was for ten nights, at a hospital that is a two-hour round trip from her home. Val recalls: 'You're so far away from your family and any support, it's a one-hour trip, and people can't just come up to see you. Tony and Thomas came up each evening, but it's not fair on Thomas.' When Mollie was in hospital recently, Chris and Tracy were not both allowed to stay with her overnight as Chris recalls: 'I had to go at 12 o'clock. We were quiet, we had the curtains drawn round the bed, I was sleeping in a chair and I was quite happy to stay in the chair, and I was asleep. Tracy was asleep on the fold-out bed, and the nurse woke me and told me I had to go.'

Healthcare Organisation

Communication and co-ordination between services is also an important factor in the provision of quality care as Debby explains: 'The developmental paediatrician is the consultant attached to the school. On our first meeting she stated that her intention is to pull everyone together, to make sure that someone is in charge of Michael's case, making sure that everyone knows what everyone else is doing and why. It is so nice after all this time to know where to go when I need something. We have not had this up until now. There have been so many consultants involved, all with their own area of specialism and no one with overall control' (Barrett 2007). As well as co-ordination between disciplines, Debby describes the problems that can occur because of arrangements or funding between health authorities: 'Because we deal with two different health authorities, this has raised a number of issues. For example, our community paediatrician wrote to the respiratory specialist at the lead centre requesting that Michael be reviewed by the ENT team there. The respiratory team cannot facilitate this. The community paediatrician therefore had to refer Michael to the local hospital, which therefore had to see Michael, decide that it can't do it, and then do a tertiary referral. However, the community paediatrician can refer to another lead centre, and the ENT surgeon from there has a clinic at the original lead centre.' This leaves Debby wondering why the community paediatrician cannot simply refer Michael to the hospital that knows him best.

The provision of facilities for young people with complex and continuing health needs in hospitals is a further concern in the quality of their healthcare experience. Often, basic facilities are lacking, causing individuals discomfort and loss of dignity. Rosemary describes her experience when trying to find changing facilities: 'I have asked on several occasions to be found somewhere where I could change Hollie or Christian's pad while visiting outpatients. I have never been successful yet. First, you have to ask a nurse if they have somewhere to be able to change the person – other patients visiting the clinic are compelled to listen in. You are frequently told that there is no facility to do this, but if you are lucky, they may have a room that is not being used with a bed in it. This does not overcome the problem of getting the person out of the chair onto the bed. To find a hoist for this? Impossible.' Rosemary explains how essential such facilities are: 'Many people with profound and multiple disabilities need someone to support them to use the toilet, or require the use of a height-adjustable changing bench where a carer can safely change their incontinence pad. They also need a hoisting system so they can be helped to transfer safely from their wheelchair to the toilet or changing bench. Those who are wheelchair users and who have to use incontinence pads are compelled to sit in their own defecation- and urine-soaked clothes until they go home because there is no alternative. The only alternative is for the carer to take their loved one to the disabled toilet, manually lift them onto the floor (which is unhygienic and usually dirty) and change their pad there. It is undignified, abusive and inhumane. Both they and we need a large accessible assistive toilet with clean bed, hoist, sling, toilet, and large wash basin with a large pedal bin for disposal of pads. The room should have enough space for a wheelchair, the person with disabilities, plus up to two carers. A hospital is a place where one would find the highest number of people with disabilities in one place, yet they do not cater for this most basic of needs.' Lack of facilities to enable children and young people to change position or be moved can also impair their medical assessment or care. For instance, Mr Hethrington describes an occasion when Lucy was taken for an outpatient scan, which could not be performed because there was no hoist available with which to transfer her to the scanner.

Summary

Children with complex and continuing health needs are likely to have a number of encounters with healthcare staff and services. The quality of the relationship which families develop with healthcare staff is very important to the quality of their child's experience and care and can significantly add to or reduce the stress of having a child with complex and continuing health needs.

A major factor in the quality of encounters with healthcare staff is respect. This includes whether staff respect families' knowledge of their child and their condition and show respect for the child and family as individuals and as a family. The quality of communication and information-giving is also vital, and staff being honest and showing respect for the family's ownership of and right to information about their child are important.

As well as individual relationships between families and healthcare staff, the organisation and planning of services is important. This includes clear lines of communication existing between staff and services, the provision of appropriate facilities for children and young people with complex and continuing health needs, and the provision of facilities and support for parents who stay with their children in hospital.

Chapter 9

Education

Children with complex and continuing health needs, like all children, are entitled to education, extending from pre-school to further and higher education. As well as assisting children to develop skills and knowledge, being a part of a learning environment can provide children with an opportunity to develop social skills and to mix with their peers. However, the opportunities for, and experiences of, education for children with complex and continuing health needs varies a great deal.

Some of the experiences which children and their parents have reported across a range of education settings are discussed in this chapter.

Pre-school Education

Pre-school education can provide children with learning opportunities and the chance of peer interaction which are equally important for children with complex and continuing health needs as for any other child. Some pre-school provision is excellent and families report that staff go out of their way to cater for their child's specific needs. For example, Helen recalls that David's nursery was, 'brilliant'. She continues: 'They knew about David, and when David was ready to go he was still on oxygen and he also had fits after which he could require resuscitation. At their own cost they had all their own staff trained to deal with this. He went for two days a week, and every year they had training and updates for the staff. They only ever asked me to come along when they were going on outings and then they asked me to come as a parent helper.' Debby also reports that, once a diagnosis of autistic spectrum disorder was made, it was possible for Michael to attend nursery at a school close to the family's home for five mornings a week with a package set up especially for him. This included a one-to-one worker, the nursery using the Picture Exchange Communication System (PECS), and the nursery staff working closely with the special needs team and speech and language therapist. The importance of good pre-school provision is illustrated by Debby's description of Michael's progress at this nursery. 'Michael really came on in leaps and bounds. There was a lot of input on communication and introducing others to him, learning to take turns and share. Michael loved going to nursery, he had an extremely enjoyable time there, and by the time he left his interaction with other children was developing to the point where he knew and recognised several of the others, and would go and try to join their chasing games' (Barrett 2007).

However, it can be difficult for children to access such opportunities for a number of reasons. As Sharon discovered, a child having mobility problems can affect their education opportunities: 'I did have a child minder when Zoë was smaller, because she was no different from any other baby. When it became evident that she couldn't walk and would have to go in a wheelchair, childminders who are working full-time can't look after disabled children because they have babies to look after and they can't give the child one-to-one care and do something else. There are no nurseries [in her area] that will take disabled children. So it's a question of putting them into nursery in a special school which is what Zoë did. She went to nursery at our local [special] school.' In other cases the problem is that the child's medical needs cannot be met by the pre-school education provider. Cheryl explains that the nursery which she had intended to use for Hannah was unable to administer her anticonvulsant medication. At the time she was having three or four seizures a day, which would have meant that Cheryl would have been called to the nursery very frequently, 'so it would have been completely pointless'.

Finding the Right School

Parents consistently identify the importance of finding the right school for their child. This not only means the right type of school, but a school with the right attitudes and values, and one that will be right for the individual child.

One of the reasons why finding the right school is so important is that the child may be unable to tell their parents if they are not happy at school or if the school is not right for them. Sharon explained, 'Zoë hasn't got the ability to say, "Mum I hate it here. It's not working." If I say, "Have you had an adult or assistant with you in all your lessons?" she won't remember. She might have had five lessons that day, and she won't be able to remember all of them to say, "I had one in two lessons, but not the third…".' The need to be able to trust the school is especially important as some parents have found that, despite mechanisms being agreed to meet their child's needs, schools are reluctant to facilitate them or may implement them in name but not consistently in practice. When David reached school age, he was still having seizures that could be life-threatening, and it was agreed that he would have one-to-one support at school. However, Helen recalls, "a couple of times I popped in because I was concerned about things David had said about being left on his own, and at one point I did have a word with the school nurse and she just dropped in, and the one-to-one support wasn't always there'.

The practicalities of finding the right education environment for a child can be difficult and time-consuming. In most cases children with complex and continuing health needs have to go through the statementing process, which Cheryl describes as 'quite lengthy'. She continues: 'In Hannah's case the report was quite accurate; the person who did the statement was really good. Hannah got into our first choice of school. We went to see a few schools and we got into the one we chose but some friends haven't. But you have so many forms and you have to make sure they would understand exactly what you mean. When you're filling in a form you have to think, "Is there any way they could misinterpret this?" I think because of my previous job I know the words to say, but if I didn't know that it would be much harder.' While Rachel is very positive about the statementing process, and sees it 'as helping us' it can mean that changes in a child's condition or needs can be slow to become officially recognised and acted upon, especially when, as in Emmy's case, the change requires two hospitals to communicate with each other and confirm their agreement to those dealing with the education statement. Rachel explains: 'Emmy has a care plan and you have to do what it says, and it says she needs oxygen. She doesn't need that in the day any more, but because her care plan says she needs it her support worker had to carry it about because it's in her care plan, because if anything happened to her and she hadn't got it, they'd be in trouble because it's in her care plan.'

It can take some time for families to find a suitable school for their child as Sharon explains: 'We started looking at senior schools for Zoë two years ago [two and a half years before Zoë was due to attend senior school]. Senior schools are very few and far between because of the inclusion policy. Now it looks as if we're going down the road, and we've got the LEA's [local education authority's] approval, that Zoë can go to a main-stream provision senior school.' Even when a school is found and approved, Sharon explains that there is still a lot of work to be done to ensure that a child's specific needs are met: 'It's trying to look at and work out the logistics of that to make sure that everything's in place for Zoë, because there are issues. She's the first one in this school to use a communi-cation aid. So it's all the rigmarole that goes with that, to make sure that the staff are trained and they know what they're doing. And it's also getting your voice as a parent heard because the LEA hold the purse strings.' Even when it appears that everything as been agreed and a child will be attend-ing a particular school with appropriate support, difficulties can still occur. Sharon provides an update on how, although everything appeared to be agreed for Zoë's secondary education, because delays occurred in the organisational processes involved, having thought that her secondary edu-cation was organised and agreed, six months later her place at that school is in doubt. Despite all their efforts to ensure their daughter receives the edu-cation experience that best meets her needs, with less than a year until she starts secondary education, Zoë's family is again in a position of uncertainty over her schooling.

The location of schools and the travel involved in getting to them is also a consideration for some children and their families. For example, the school that David eventually attended as a sixth former was one which the family considered when he was younger, but, because he requires assisted ventilation when he sleeps, at that time the journey was a contraindication. Helen explains, 'at that point we didn't think he would cope with the journey at the end of the day'. In some cases, because of the location of schools, enabling their child to attend the right school entails upheaval for the whole family. Simon's family has recently had to organise his second-ary education, which has meant them moving home. Judy explains that although there is a local school which he could attend, 'we're not very happy with that and we don't want him to go there so we're moving'.

The nature of children's needs may mean that it is not always clear whether they fit the entry criteria for a given school. Helen explains that the school nurse at David's school suggested they seek a sixth form place for him at a school for children with medical problems. 'Although he has got a specific medical problem, I wasn't sure that he met the criteria. But the school nurse said, "Well, why not call them?" So I rang to the headmaster and he was great. He said David met the criteria.'

As Helen explains, it is not always easy to tell, on a one-off visit, whether a school will be right for an individual child. Helen describes how one school that they visited assisted in this process by enabling David to spend some time there alone before making his decision. 'We came away [after visiting the school together] and we said to David, "What do you think?" And he said, "I did like it but I'd like to spend some more time there." So we telephoned the headmaster and asked if David could go back again, without us, and he said, yes, bring him for a day. So we took him, dropped him off, picked him up, and he said he wanted to go there.'

As well as the time and effort required, Rosemary recalls the emotional impact of seeking schools for Christian and Hollie: 'I went round to a couple of schools, and I walked out of sobbing one of them. It would appear that the highest goal they expected the young children to levitate to was to look at a mobile and reach out to touch it. No appreciation that the child might be functioning at beyond a few weeks of age. The demeaning attitude that they had. The children had their coats on at two o'clock, waiting to go home at quarter past three. I said, "Why have they got their coats on?" And it was, "Oh, it takes a long time to get their coats on."'

Schools

Children with complex and continuing health needs access education in a range of settings, including mainstream schools and special schools. Siobhan attends a mainstream school, and Evelyn is very pleased with how the arrangements for this have been handled. She had no problem getting Siobhan into mainstream school and describes how her experiences have led her to conclude that, as well as the benefits to Siobhan, the benefits of inclusion for society in general are significant. 'Inclusion is fantastic, because when I think back to my own childhood there was a special needs school near us, and I think of how scared we were of those kids, and some of them were probably just like Siobhan, it breaks my heart. I know children in our school ridiculed them.' She describes how she hopes that with greater inclusion and openness the ignorance which breeds prejudice will be reduced.

In contrast, Helen and David's experience of trying to access mainstream education for David was not positive. At the time of his transition to middle school, David and his parents looked at mainstream and special school options. At one mainstream school, a school that the family would have favoured, they found the headmaster's attitude to David and his needs very negative. Helen recalls: 'We went there and he said, "You won't get one-to-one support for him. That won't happen," even though it was funded by the health authority and there was no indication that they were going to stop it. He just said, "You won't get that, it just doesn't happen at middle school." It was almost as if, because he felt like that, we didn't want to go there. It was awful, it was a really good school. It gets really good results but we came away thinking, "I don't want my child to go there if that's their attitude to him."' After their negative experience at the mainstream school, David's family looked at a special school. In contrast to their previous experience, the headmaster at this school was very positive about David having one-to-one support: 'We said that he has had one-to-one support and we would like that to continue, and he said, "You'll be lucky, because we have classes of ten with two staff, but I am quite happy to support you." So he made it a condition that David would be accepted at the school if he had one-to-one support, and he got it.'

In other instances, although individual staff may be very supportive, processes or regulations make it difficult for children to access mainstream education. Rachel is very impressed with the headmaster at the school which Emmy will attend (the school which her other daughters attend) and recalls that he was very supportive of her going there. However, Rachel explains that other factors have made Emmy's attendance problematic. 'Initially, the school was really good about it. The nurses went to the school to deal with the oxygen, and made sure that they know what they've got to do if she has an apnoea.' However, 'all of a sudden, just before Emmy started school it was delayed because someone had gone to the union about it and the union had said no, you can't touch this child.

You can't take her.' Rachel explains that the person who will be Emmy's classroom support assistant is 'absolutely brilliant…if I went to her and said, "Emmy needs this" she'd say, "Oh fine, show me how to do it" but she's not a member of the union, because she's not actually a teacher. The headmaster said he was really sorry but he would have to delay Emmy starting because they have to have a back-up, because if the classroom support assistant broke her leg and Emmy had an apnoea at the same time, they wouldn't have any cover.' Eventually, the headmaster was the only other person willing to take responsibility for Emmy, so he will now act as her back-up.

Sometimes parents find that mainstream education is not the right thing for the individual child because they will not be truly included with the other pupils. When Michael was old enough to start school, it transpired that a mainstream school would have to write an entire curriculum just for him and he would spend a considerable amount of each day on his own with a teacher. Debby explains: 'Our concern was that we didn't want him in a mainstream school where he was singled out as "different". He wouldn't have benefited.' Instead, the family found a special school which met Michael's needs and where he would be included with his peers throughout the school day. For Michael, this has been the best option and Debby describes his school as 'really good, they get the most out of him and get him to achieve his potential'.

Where schools are familiar with and confident in supporting children with complex and continuing health medical needs it can significantly enhance the opportunities which they have to participate in a range of activities. One contrast that David and his parents have found since he attends a school for children with physical and medical problems is, 'this school is used to dealing with very complex medical things, whereas his previous school wasn't used to the medical needs, they were more learning difficulties'. This means that the school does not let David's medical needs stand in the way of him participating in the activities that he wants to engage in. Helen recalls: 'They went camping and the person organising it rang me and said, "We're going camping. What do we need to do to make this possible for David?" There was no question of can he do it, it was: he's doing it, and what do we have to do to make it happen safely? And it happened.'

However, in some cases children are not best catered for in schools that appear, on paper, to meet their needs most closely. Because Rosemary is aware of Christian's intelligence, she arranged, with great difficulty, for him to attend a school for children with physical disabilities rather than a school for children with learning disabilities. However, 'Christian hated it. He used to come home upset day after day after day. Really upset.' In order to try to find out what the problem was, Rosemary would go to the school unannounced. She found that 'time after time Christian was excluded. I really let rip when I walked in and all the children were sitting at the tables doing maths with their exercise books, but Christian was in the corner underneath the table with a mobile. I said, "Where is Christian? Where is his exercise book?" and I was told, "Well, he doesn't have one, he doesn't do maths." So we took him out and he went to a school that is noted as a school of excellence within the learning disabilities field.'

Complex Needs

One issue related to the education that is available for children with complex and continuing health needs may be whether their medical or technical interventions can be managed while they are at school. Val considers Catherine's school to be excellent and hugely supportive not only of Catherine but of the family as a whole. 'Catherine's pre-school years were really difficult, her reflux was so bad that she was constantly having chest infections from aspirated vomit, which required urgent hospitalisation for oxygen and steroids. Her mainstream nursery found this very difficult to cope with. She had a nasogastric tube at this time, which was often pulled out by the other children, and I had to go in and repass it for her. I only worked two mornings a week but it was all so stressful I came very close to giving up work to be able to respond when they needed help. It was like a breath of fresh air when she started at her special school. They are so experienced and able to take control of things, they were looking to support me rather than vice versa.' However, this level of support is not always available at schools. Although the headmaster of the school that Emmy will attend is very positive about her going there, Rachel explains that her medical and technical needs have been an issue. She will need a gastrostomy feed while she is at school, and no one will be available to give this. The headmaster would be willing to do so, but will often be unavailable at lunchtime owing to meetings and other commitments. The class-room support assistant cannot give the feed as she is legally required to have a lunch break. Rachel could go into school and give the feed, but this has been deemed inappropriate: 'They say that other parents don't come in at dinner time, so why should hers. But I said she is entitled to a feed. So I contacted [a boy with a gastrostomy's] Mum, and asked her how she did it, and she said that he comes out and I feed him. But the hospital have advised the school that that's not an option because they want to make Emmy's school day as normal as possible.' However, Rachel feels that this would be the best option, because, as she explains, 'not having a feed is not normal. They said she can miss a feed and I can put more on her overnight feed so she's still getting the same calories, but I think that's not a normal thing. If we want normal, that's not a normal situation.'

In some cases a school's provision for children with complex and con-tinuing health needs means that they have to miss schooling when there is no medical need for this. Lucy needs a nurse to be on site at her school when she is present because she requires regular medication, may need additional medication, and sometimes oxygen, if she has a seizure. This can mean that Lucy has to miss school for reasons not directly related to her own day-to-day health. For example, one year there was a heavy snowfall that prevented the school nurse getting to school, which meant that Lucy could not go to school although she was well enough to attend and able to get in.

Transition to Further or Higher Education

When a young person with complex and continuing health needs is ready to progress to further or higher education, effecting this transition can present a challenge. This may be because of the lack of transitional arrangements for a child who has been used to small classes and one-to-one support, and who is suddenly faced with large classes with little support. Helen explains how David was reluctant to go to a large mainstream college for his sixth form years, 'because this college has got hundreds and hundreds of people, and he was used to a small school, being in a class of ten, with one-to-one support, and he was suddenly expected to go to this college where there were thousands of people. He didn't want one-to-one support any more, but he couldn't cope with that. It was too big a leap.' Helen also describes how having a transition period can make a vast difference to the young person's ability to progress. David has spent his first year of sixth form in a school with small classes but without one-to-one support and with more autonomy. 'We are thinking of, possibly, him going to the college that he didn't want to go to before, because he is used to having less support now. He has become a lot more independent and has increased his confidence.' Although, as Helen explains, David was ready to move away from the intensity of one-to-one support, the transition to a complete absence of support in a large and impersonal environment was too great for a single step, 'because, as much as his one-to-one could drive him mad being there all the time, he did get a bit worried if she wasn't there. At this school, they have let him go. The teacher said to me at his review, "We try to let David do things as independently as possible. We know where he is *most* of the time." And I said, "I don't want to know that!" But I think that has been good and he is gaining confidence and he is thinking that he might go to the other college and we're going to their open day to have a look round.' David confirms that he has enjoyed his new school and the greater level of independence which it allows him. He is a keen sportsman, and is interested in doing sports and leisure at the college.

Enabling a young person with complex and continuing health needs to secure a place in further education can sometimes be beset with practical and organisational problems, especially if they have multiple needs and communication problems. In Christian's case, in order for him to go to college the professionals involved in his education had to compile a report because the Learning Skills Council will only fund ongoing education if it can see progression. The educational psychologist who compiled the report described Christian as functioning at a cognitive level of age two to three months. Rosemary comments: 'How someone, who does not know a person, who probably has only just been introduced to them, can go through their standard assessment sheet, ticking and crossing appropriate boxes, then declare what their level of understanding is, is beyond all reason. The person being assessed, quite understandably, will object to a complete stranger entering their life and expecting tasks to be completed and performed like a trained dog. No appreciation is given to relationship-building between them. No acceptance that the person may be having ill health during this "half-hour session", or what the side effects may be of any medication they may have been given.' The assessment result was not only at stark odds with what Rosemary knows Christian's abilities to be, but also presented the practical problem of whether the Learning Skills Council would fund Christian's further education. Fortunately, the family has a good friend who is the one of the heads of inclusive education at a university. Rosemary invited him, as a friend, to Christian's final review and recalls, 'he took up this educational psychologist's report and completely pulled it to shreds and humiliated her and tore her off such a strip, and just about everybody else in the room. It is lucky for her that she, once again, was unable to attend the review. The people in the room were so speechless and humiliated themselves that they could hardly speak.' With this report overturned, Christian is now happily settled in Beaumont College, North Lancaster, where the staff are very pleased with his progress as Rosemary explains: 'They fully appreciate that he can read, he gets the credit he is due, and he has had to reach 19 years of age before he can be in an education establishment that treats him as a human being.'

Even when funding for further education is approved, if the young person's health makes attendance problematic securing funding to afford them the opportunity to gain exposure to education that equals that of their peers may be problematic. Despite making good progress at college, Christian's health problems and the need to attend a variety of appointments have meant that he has missed a great deal of college time during his first three years. Although the college is very supportive of him being offered the opportunity to remain for an extra year, to catch up on this time, finding funding for this and convincing the Learning Skills Council of its worth has involved considerable work for Rosemary.

Summary

Children with complex and continuing health needs should be afforded equal opportunities to access education as any other child. The ideal is that this should be provided in a mainstream education environment, and in a manner which truly includes and values the child. Although some families report that accessing mainstream education has been relatively unproblematic and a very positive experience, there are also instances where this has not been the case. This may be because of organisational issues, the attitudes of individuals and organisations, and the reality that the 'inclusion' offered will not truly allow the child to be included with their peers.

The differences in education provision for children with complex and continuing health needs can begin at pre-school level, with some families reporting high quality provision, whereas others struggle to find appropriate pre-school education for their children. When children reach school age, there are again significant variations in the provision available. These may be related to the attitudes of staff at schools, practicalities related to provision, or whether or not a child will be truly included and enabled to participate in the range of education opportunities, including socialisation and interaction with peers. The child's medical and technical needs, and the provision of support for these in schools also affects the child's attendance and ability to engage in a full range of learning experiences.

When a child reaches the age at which further education is appropriate, this can create additional challenges, such as provision for a transition to the further education environment and the assessment processes involved in determining whether funding will be made available.

Chapter 10

Society

The attitude of society towards children with complex and continuing health needs is an important factor in the quality of life that children and their families enjoy and the opportunities which children are afforded. This includes how individuals respond to children and their families, and how society and services are organised. Children and their families report some very positive and some very negative experiences, some instances where provision is excellent and others where it is very poor. Some of these experiences and how they affect the lives of individuals and families are described in this chapter.

Facilities for Children and their Families

The provision of facilities that can be used by children with complex and continuing health needs and their families is very important in the quality of their lives. The quality of provision affects the activities that children and their families can engage in, and the opportunities which they have as individuals and as families. Rosemary highlights one example of excellence in this respect, not just for the facilities provided but also because of the attitudes of the staff who work there, the Trafford Centre in Manchester. She describes a shopping trip with Christian and Hollie. 'When we had to go for something to eat we could not find a table big enough for two wheelchairs plus three adults. Being a Saturday and edging towards Christmas, the place was packed. I asked a guide to help us find a table. Having circled the whole of the eating area, none could be found. So, what did she do? Perfect solution, and one that I will always remember. The guide took us to one side where there was enough empty space, summoned two extra assistants, and brought a table to us, together with chairs. Now there's service.' In contrast, many families report poor provision of facilities for them to go shopping with their children as Sharon explains: 'There's only one supermarket in Basingstoke that I can go to, and that's Asda because it's the only one that has disabled children's trolleys. Other stores are meant to have them but they've all gone for a walk.' Other aspects of shopping can also be beset with problems. Sharon describes how, 'if Zoë wants new clothes I have to buy three sizes and bring them home because the changing rooms aren't actually set up for disabled people. Very few of them have seats, very few of them have rails. And they're not always big enough to put a wheelchair in, either. If I've got to go shopping for me, I'm not going to leave her outside the changing room, and I don't necessarily want to leave the door wide open so I can keep an eye on Zoë. The disabled changing room at British Home Stores is usually full of stock. I've said to them, "This is a disabled changing room, why is it full of stock?" and the answer is "That's where we've been told to put it." Also, a lot of the aisles are so close together that if you push Zoë down an aisle all the clothes come off [the displays].' Chris and Tracy also cite a large shopping centre in a nearby town where there are no lifts to the upper shopping mall. As Chris explains: 'You don't think about it until you've got oxygen and a buggy that is sturdy enough to take the oxygen, and you can't get upstairs unless you are able to carry the baby, the oxygen and the buggy.'

Accessing suitable toilets and changing facilities is often a major issue for disabled children and their families. Again, the Trafford Centre in Manchester is cited as an example of high-quality provision in this respect. Cheryl and Steve explain that this is one of the few places in the country that has changing facilities that are suitable for children. Rosemary describes them: 'We were greeted with a large room, big enough for the disabled person and their chair, enough for two carers (plus even more) to move about freely. Not only was there a clean, height-adjustable bench with a large blue paper roll – but a remarkably smooth overhead three-dimensional tracking hoist together with a multi-adjustable sling, toilet, large wash hand basin, and big bin. It was terrific! If not for this, we would have had no alternative but to return home early.' However, in other locations, the provision of changing facilities is very poor as Sharon recalls: 'Zoë is dry now, but she wasn't, and apart from baby changing stations, there is nowhere around, not even at the hospital, that has changing benches. So we used to have to, as a friend of mine does whose son is 12, take a changing mat, and put it on a toilet floor to change the child, because there is no facility. I have never yet been anywhere where there is a facility. But who wants to put their child on a filthy floor to change their nappy? Or they do it on the back seat of the car.'

Where a child requires assisted feeding, there are rarely facilities that enable families to do this with any degree of privacy. Debby explains the conundrum of where to carry out Michael's gastrostomy feeds when they are out: 'Mother and baby rooms, or in public, to looks and stares that set him out as different?'

As well as the availability of practical facilities, organisations and individuals enabling children to be included in the usual range of family commemorations is important. However, sometimes apparently unnecessary regulations from companies or individuals make this impossible as Cheryl recalls when she took Hannah for a Pixie Foto: 'Because Hannah couldn't sit up, they wouldn't take a photo. We ended up having proper photos done in the end, which are really nice, but because she couldn't sit up they wouldn't do it. They wouldn't take her photo lying down, because at her age she should have been sitting up.'

Leisure Activities

As highlighted in Chapter 2, children with complex and continuing health needs have the same right to play and enjoyment as other children, and the provision of play and leisure facilities for them and their families is therefore important. However, the availability of such facilities is variable as Sharon recalls: 'We went to a friend's house in Farnborough during half-term, and they actually have a disabled playground near where they live. Fantastic. The slide had a ramp, so Zoë used her walker, got to the top, put her walker down, slid to the bottom, I met her, and we went round again. They have roundabouts you can put wheelchairs on, they've got this big spider net that the child can lie on as a swing. So it's set up so non-able and able children can use them.' However, such facilities are not universally available. Sharon contrasts how, closer to home, 'there's nothing in Basingstoke that's suitable for disabled children. We can take Zoë to the park across the road, but I've got to have the energy to take her, and I can't get on half the stuff. It's not disabled friendly, so it's OK if you can get on them with them, or go round with them, but otherwise you've had it.' As well as the lack of facilities for individual children, provision of facilities that allow integration of disabled and able-bodied children is important as Sharon explains: 'If you've got siblings you don't always want to home in on special needs all the time. You want to try and integrate with everyone else, but often you can't do it.' Judy also describes how finding activities that Simon and his brothers can all engage in is almost impossible. Simon likes to go swimming, but this tends to be restricted to him going with his school because of the difficulty of getting him in and out of the pool, and the risk of him having a seizure while he is swimming.

Sometimes families find that the facilities for disabled children are not appropriate even when they are apparently provided for them, as Sharon explains: 'If I want to take Zoë to the cinema, the disabled seats are about four feet from the screen, right at the front under the screen. Then they've got stairs all the way up the middle. So I have to take her out of her chair and walk her up the stairs because she can't sit in the front because it's too big and too loud. Having to sit right at the front you miss half of what goes on and you're straining your neck because it's too close. Why they've put them at the front I don't know, but there are 12 screens and it's the same in every one.'

Transport

The provision of transport facilities is also important for children and their families. Within this, a major issue for many families is the provision of parking facilities. Families frequently report an apparent lack of recognition that having a young disabled child creates a specific need. Chris and Tracy describe how it took 'a lot of fighting' for them to be permitted to have a disabled parking bay outside their house. This seems to be because access to disabled parking facilities does not come into effect until a child is three years old. Tracy and Chris eventually contacted their MP, and a representative from the council was required to visit the family to assess Mollie and determine whether the family needed a disabled parking bay. Chris recalls: 'This woman walked in the door and said, "I don't know why I'm here. I can see she needs it!" We had oxygen bottles, oxygen tubing…but if you just put that in writing to them, the criteria is three years old. She's under three. Sorry.'

Debby describes how difficult transporting a child who is oxygen-dependent can be, especially when access to disabled parking facilities are denied them: 'Oxygen cylinders are really heavy and bulky, but you're not entitled to a disabled parking sticker under the age of two, because "they don't walk under age two anyway". So you have to park in a regular parking space. The oxygen cylinder is heavy and bulky, and it is attached to Michael. The grey bag goes over your shoulder or under the pushchair but you've only got a certain amount of lead, and the oxygen has to be on Michael, so it all has to be taken out at once. Michael, oxygen, and buggy, and you don't have space to do that. And as you lean forwards the oxygen slips off your shoulder. And you also have two other children.' Chris explains that as well as the practicalities of parking and getting equipment in and out of the car, they were not permitted to use disabled parking facilities when Mollie was oxygen-dependent. 'My main concern was, what if we have to get her back to the hospital quickly, and then we have to park a few streets away, and carry her and her oxygen for a few streets, when she isn't well.'

As well as regulations related to families accessing disabled parking facilities, individual attitudes can cause them problems, as Cheryl recalls: 'We have a disabled badge, and if I am taking Philipa and Hannah I have double buggy. So I pulled up in a disabled bay with my disabled badge and once a guy said to me, "This isn't mother and baby parking you know." And I just said, "And can a child not be disabled?" but he just saw a mother putting two children in a buggy.' Similarly, Chris and Tracy have found that despite obtaining the disabled bay outside their house, this is not respected by other motorists. Tracy explains: 'We got the disabled bay on Monday and by Wednesday someone had parked in it. I think they see us and think "They don't need it" and so they use it.' Chris recalls: 'We had someone who told me to F*** off. I went up to them and said, very politely, "This is a disabled bay and it's here for a reason." And he said, "That's not my problem. F*** off."' Another motorist left his car parked in the bay for two days. Tracy left a note on it explaining that this was a disabled bay and asking him to move. She explains: 'I left a note on his car, it wasn't a horrible note, just explaining, and he and his wife knocked on our door, and he said "Did you leave a note on my car?" and I said "Yes" and he said

"Well, don't you think that's a bit out of order?" and I said, "Don't you think it's out of order parking in a disabled bay? We've got a disabled child." And he said, "Oh, I didn't know that."'

There are also often limitations on children with complex and continuing health needs and their families using public transport. Sharon describes how, even when facilities for people with disabilities exist on public transport, these are often unreliable. 'We can't go on public transport because some of the buses have got drop steps but some haven't, and you can't guarantee which you'll get. So we rely on the car. It's a motobility car and we rely on the car and that's it. But if we wanted to use public transport we'd have problems.' Similarly, Sharon explains that the facilities provided on trains for passengers with disabilities are not reliable. 'Trains have only got a few disabled places and when they've gone you can't get on. But you can't book a place. So it could be a case of we're all going up to London for the day and we get to the station and we can't go. You try explaining that to a child who's got special needs at the best of times, "Why can't we go? I don't understand."'

Sharon explains how even if the family manages to get to London by train, the capital city's transport does not really cater for people with disabilities. 'If you go up to London you've got to watch where you go because you can't use all the Underground stations. Because it's all stairs and escalators, and you can't put wheelchairs on those…or, if you do, they don't like it! So the only way is one of us carrying her and one of us collapsing the wheelchair, which you can do, but it's a bit of a rigmarole. So it's a case of once you get out of Waterloo you have to take a taxi because most of the taxis take wheelchairs, because it's the only way you can get to where you need to go.' Like so many other aspects of having a child with complex and continuing health needs, this means that a family day out attracts more expense than it would for another child.

Individual Responses

Parents report that as well as the variable quality of facilities for their children, the attitude and behaviour which other people exhibit towards them varies greatly. Rosemary generally finds individual people's responses to Christian and Hollie quite positive, even when she is performing medical or technical procedures on them: 'People either take no notice or they might just come and ask what I'm doing, and it sometimes turns out they have a relative in hospital having tube feeds and they just want to know if it would help them.' Rosemary also recalls how some comments take her by surprise, because although they are made about her children, they bypass their disabilities. 'One time I was out with Hollie, and I had all the suction equipment and everything on her chair. Hollie hates wearing shoes, and she spends all her time trying to get them off by rubbing her feet on her footplate. So, eventually I took them off, and this woman said to her friend, "Oh, look at that poor child. Her mother can't afford any shoes." Nothing about the equipment, or the chair, just her shoes.'

However, some families also report people giving negative or intrusive responses to their children. This is often unintentional, as Chris explains: 'There is a lot of prejudice, and also people who just don't think. I was probably like that before. If you haven't had that experience, you don't always think.' Nevertheless, such attention can be offensive or insulting to children and their families. Tracy recalls: 'When Mollie was on oxygen, I know it's only human, but people did a double-take, and that really annoyed me. That's my baby, don't stare at us.' Val reports how this level of unwanted observation can affect the whole family. She describes an occasion when the family was returning from holiday on a ferry and she had to feed Catherine using her gastrojejunostomy tube: 'At one point Thomas was reading his book and he went under the seat and I said "What are you doing under there?" and he said, "I'm fed up of those people staring at us." There was a family opposite staring at us the whole time, while I did the feed and everything.' Sharon also explains, 'If Zoë is in her wheelchair they can see she is different, but she doesn't look disabled. It doesn't bother me as much as it did. Zoë never takes any notice, but her sister sometimes says, "They're staring at her again."'

Sometimes families find that the observation to which they are subjected includes a judgemental element. Sharon recounts her experiences of having Zoë in the seat of her shopping trolley at Asda, 'The amount of stares you get from people is unbelievable. Because...well, she's a big child, what is she doing sat in there? It's also the stares that you get when you have a child who suddenly goes through a temper tantrum and screams and shouts. "Well, you ought to control that child." Or the stares when you're at the doctor's surgery and she gets out of her wheelchair and she bunny hops round. You can tell that she's nearly ten, the stares, and the

"Why isn't she walking?" Sometimes I will say something if I can then get up and walk out, but if I've then got to sit in that situation I won't say anything.' Debby also describes how, although some leisure parks such as Legoland have a system by which disabled guests can be given bands to exempt them from queuing, if they use these, the family can be 'looked at for jumping queues'. She explains that people will rarely if ever ask them why they have done this, so they do not have a chance to explain, they are just aware of the silent accusing stares. Similarly, if Michael goes into 'meltdown' they have to endure the unspoken but blatant criticism of onlookers.

Rachel also describes the intrusive and insulting responses which people sometimes make to her children: 'I can't be doing with people who say, "What's wrong with her [Emmy]?" There was this woman in town going to her daughter, "That baby has only got one eye, I wonder what's wrong with it" and I thought, "I'm not going to say anything because I'll only say something I'll regret." But she was going on and saying, "Come here and look at it. It's only got one eye." In the end I went to her and said, "It is a she and your daughter is going to end up as ignorant as you. There's nothing wrong with her. She happened to be born with a facial deformity. Nothing happened." If people say to me, "What's wrong with her?" I say, "Why, what's up?" and they say, "Well, her eye…" and I say, "Oh, that, no there's nothing wrong. She just has a blind eye. I thought you meant something had happened to her."'

In some cases families have noted that a specific event has increased public scrutiny of them and their children. Cheryl and Steve report a marked difference in how Hannah is looked at by strangers since she has begun to use a wheelchair. Cheryl describes how, 'up until she got her wheelchair on her second birthday nobody batted an eyelid at her. You could walk down the street with her in a buggy and nobody would look at her or give her a second thought. Nobody did a double-take. We got a wheelchair on her second birthday and we went to the Trafford Centre and people were turning round, and we noticed it straight away. I was heavily pregnant as well and you could see people look at her, and then look at my bump and then, oh, sympathy. You could see it all over their faces. It was really weird.'

Children and their families are also sometimes subjected to thoughtless comments. These can be, as Evelyn explains, comments that, to the user, are just, 'words that are thrown about, but to someone else they are the worst insult that you can ever give'. For example, she recalls: 'If my daughter came home and said that someone called someone a spastic at school, I used to take it so personally, that word, because my daughter's got cerebral palsy. I used to say, "Bring those people to me, ask them if they know what that word means."' In addition, Evelyn describes how, although such incidents are relatively infrequent, occasionally the comments that others make without thinking can have a long-lasting effect on children and their families. Although Siobhan can walk, because she gets very tired, she has a special buggy which she uses when necessary. Evelyn recalls, 'I had Siobhan and Devin in a double buggy and we went into a shop and the security guard said to Siobhan, not even to me' "You're too big to be in that pram."' Again, when Siobhan was in her buggy, 'an old man come up to her and said to her, "You're too big to be in that buggy."' Evelyn explains, 'since the old man incident, we've probably only used the buggy when Siobhan is ill, because she refuses to go in it'. The result of this thoughtless comment is that Evelyn, Siobhan and her siblings are restricted in what they can do because Siobhan is embarrassed to use her buggy, but becomes exhausted if she attempts to walk long distances. As Evelyn explains: 'These people make comments and walk away. They forget about it, but you're left with it.'

Sometimes it is not negative responses *per se*, but inappropriately positive feedback that can be very condescending or insulting to children. Sharon explains: 'When Zoë uses her talking aid in a mainstream environment, everybody will suddenly clap, but why? Because she's only talking. Why are you doing that? She's only talking, like a ten-year-old would. That is her voice. That's how she communicates. You wouldn't clap a ten-year-old for talking. But that's what happens. I don't mind people saying, "Well done, that looked difficult to use." That's different, but to clap and say, "That was absolutely brilliant."' Cheryl also notes that Hannah being so beautiful and not immediately striking one as disabled means that some people have said to her, 'but she's so pretty. She looks so normal.' Cheryl comments that, although this is intended as a compliment, it indicates a concern about their views on disability, as she explains: 'Yes, she does. But does that mean she doesn't have a disability?'

Rosemary illustrates the vast spectrum of individuals' responses to her children by recounting an occasion on which she encountered very positive and extremely negative behaviour from individuals at the same time. 'I think the worst thing we had was at Lourdes. We were at the grotto. The Spanish and Italians were trying to push us out of the way at the grotto. They were so rude, they were literally pushing us, and stepping over the wheelchair, pushing the wheelchair out of the way so that they could get to the front. As we were being pushed and shoved, a few yards into the grotto, crushed against the wall was a Japanese father and daughter. They had politely stood aside to accommodate the swelling masses of people. It was not in their nature to push themselves forwards. The father and daughter saw us in our plight. No words were spoken, but our eyes met and true understanding "without using words to communicate" were exchanged. With a gentle and graceful nod of the head, the father then stood his ground and parted the throngs of pushing forceful "tourists" (not pilgrims) out of the way so that we were able to untangle the wheels of Hollie and Christian's wheelchairs from the shoes, feet, and legs of others who thought that their needs outstripped anyone else. We were forced along with the tidal flow of people behind us so I was unable to nod my appreciation to him. Of all the things we saw and did on our visit to Lourdes, that moment, and the kindness that man showed, will be the most vivid.'

Summary

The attitudes that children with complex and continuing health needs and their families encounter in society are a significant influence on the quality of their lives. This can include the way in which services and facilities are organised and the way in which individual people respond to them.

There is clearly the potential for everyday facilities to be made accessible and user-friendly for children and their families, including shopping, eating, toilet and changing facilities. However, unfortunately, examples of high-quality provision in these respects are very limited. The provision of play and leisure facilities is another area where facilities and access varies, but where high-quality provision makes a great difference not only to the child but to the whole family.

Public transport facilities are sometimes suitable for children with complex and continuing health needs to use. However, the variability and unreliability of such provision can make using public transport almost impossible for families. Although this means that families often have no alternative but to rely on using a car, parking facilities can also be problematic for them, particularly when their child is very young.

As well as the provision of facilities, the attitudes and responses that children receive from individuals are important and can affect the self-image or self-perception of the child, their siblings and family. Negative responses from individuals, as well as the availability of physical facilities, can significantly affect on whether children and their families can enjoy activities together.

Chapter 11

Working with Children and their Families

In the previous chapters of this book we have explored the experiences of children who have complex and continuing health needs and their families. In this chapter the experiences of health and social care staff who support children and their families on a day-to-day basis are discussed. This discussion includes staff who support children and their families in their own homes, and those who work in residential settings.

Working with children and their families can be very satisfying, but can also present staff with a number of challenges. This chapter describes some of the realities of working with children and their families.

Staff and Organisations

The following staff and organisations have contributed to this chapter. Some have agreed to their real names being used while some have chosen to use pseudonyms.

CHASE Hospice Care for Children – Christopher's: Tania

Tania trained as a nursery nurse and has worked on the community team at Christopher's Hospice (a part of CHASE Children's Hospice Care for Children) for four and a half years. This team provides families whose children have life-limiting illnesses, complex care needs, or whom require palliative care with respite care in their own homes. The time and frequency of respite care varies according to the family's needs. Tania previously worked in a hospital, and also with a child who required long-term assisted ventilation at home.

The Children's Trust at Tadworth: Sue, Claire, Mary, Kate and Fiona

The Children's Trust at Tadworth is a national charity that works with children who have multiple disabilities and complex health needs, their families and other carers. The Trust offers a range of services, including short-, medium- and long-term residential care; therapy; rehabilitation; transitional care; and short breaks (either on-site or in the family home). The Trust also offers education, care and therapy for children and young people at St Margaret's School.

Sue manages outreach services at The Children's Trust. The outreach team provide families with support in their own homes, either while they are present, or by caring for the child while the family leaves the home for a period. Primary care trusts purchase this service from The Children's Trust when they are not able to provide it themselves. Sue has previously held a similar post in a primary care trust.

Claire works as a site co-ordinator at The Children's Trust. She has previously worked in paediatric intensive care units, in the community, and on the outreach team at The Children's Trust. The site co-ordinators provide on-site support for staff as they take on more and more complex caseloads, and they provide a significant education and training input for all staff.

Mary, Kate and Fiona work with children who need long-term residential care. This includes children who require rehabilitation and children who are cared for at The Children's Trust until the right place is found for them to live.

Clinovia Ltd

Clinovia Ltd is an experienced community-based healthcare provider. The company supports the National Health Service, social and educational organisations by providing tailored home healthcare. One area that Clinovia specialises in is providing care to individuals with complex care needs. The company is currently commissioned by a number of primary care trusts to provide support for children and their families.

Several staff who work for Clinovia's complex care team have contributed to this book. These include seven healthcare support workers, who provide families with the day-to-day support needed to enable their child to live at home, two nurse co-ordinators, whose role is primarily managerial and related to a specific caseload which can include children and adults, one lead nurse (lead nurses each cover a specific geographical area and have management responsibility for all the teams in that area).

Griffin House: Val

Val and Dave own Griffin House Children's Home. Dave is employed by the local social services department and Val was previously the children's services manager at a neighbouring local authority. They decided to open a small children's home which could concentrate on providing high-quality support that places families centrally in the child's life.

Working with Children

Many staff describe the privilege and responsibility that being entrusted with the care for other people's children carries. One of the Clinovia team comments, 'parents are putting their child in your hands, trusting you to look after them'. Val also explains, '[it is] a privilege to be given the opportunity to look after someone else's child and for the parents to place that level of trust in us'.

Despite the responsibility which it entails, staff describe the overwhelming reward of their work as being the children with whom they work. As Fiona explains, 'it's just the children'. The rewards that being with the children bring include getting to know the children as individuals, understanding their characters, and their likes and dislikes. One of the healthcare support workers from Clinovia describes the pleasures of her work: 'You play with the child. You get to know about their character.' Fiona comments that it is not only her getting to know the children, but the children getting to know, bond with, and respond to her that is rewarding. This is not solely because of the relationship which develops between the child and member of staff, so that, as Kate describes, 'they are like a part of you', but being able to understand and respond to the child's cues and needs. Despite the reward which it brings, achieving this can be challenging, especially when a child has difficulty in communicating. Mary explains: 'You learn to read the children. If they haven't got the formal communication skills to be able to say "I've got a pain here, I'm not happy, I'm uncomfortable" you have to go through a communication process, and because you know them, you can usually work out what's wrong with them and solve those problems.'

Mary clarifies the importance of remembering when deducing what each child wants to communicate that, despite the child's specific needs, 'they are children, they can have all the usual things that children can have, or they might just be fed up'. As this illustrates, a part of knowing a child is seeing beyond their medical or technical needs to the person whom they are, and engaging with them as an individual. One of the nurse co-ordinators from Clinovia describes how working closely with children and their families allows her the satisfaction of 'doing that holistic nursing–looking at every aspect of their life'. Although staff appreciate the importance of meeting children's medical or technical needs, seeing the whole child and attempting to assist or support them in every aspect of their lives is seen equally as a vital part of their work. For example, Claire comments that one of the satisfying aspects of her work is being able to spend time helping children to find and participate in activities which they enjoy, enabling them to play and have fun, rather than focusing primarily on their medical or technical needs. Mary also explains, 'you go out into the big wide world and see the social side of their needs as well'.

Despite the rewards of working with and getting to know children, their needs can present staff with some very practical challenges as Val describes how: 'Two of the young people we have with us at the moment have cri-du-chat syndrome, which means that they cannot speak, are doubly incontinent, and function at about two to four years of age although they are 16 with the usual hormones and pre-menstrual tension that other 16-year-olds have. The working shifts last for 14 hours so that there is continuity for the children in that the person who sees them off to school is there when they come home and at bedtime. The staff do not get a minute to themselves as the children are into everything in the way that toddlers are, the children may bite, hit, kick, and so on, and if distressed will self-harm. The job is both mentally and physically exhausting.'

Being a part of the process and the team which enables children to be cared for in the 'right place' can be a significant source of reward for staff. In some cases, this can be because they play a part in enabling a child to be cared for at home. As one of the healthcare support workers, from Clinovia comments: 'I looked after a little boy who was in hospital for three years before he eventually went home. The difference was amazing really. I saw how much difference it made when he went home. How much he improved. The girl I work with now, she's at home, and at college. Living her life, like she should do. She should do that, she's 17 and she has every right to that.' Another healthcare support worker describes how 'the first baby I worked with was 11 months old before he came out of hospital, and when he got home, his parents' faces just lit up and he was there with his family, and the family could all come round and visit, so it was just their home environment, they were so happy to have him back. It was a real achievement for them, and for me to be there with them.' The reward of seeing a child in the right place for them and their family can apply equally to them being provided with appropriate residential care, as Val explains, 'seeing a child settle into placement, laugh and flourish is a reward in itself'.

Working with the Family

Many staff describe their role in supporting parents and other family members as equally rewarding as working with the children themselves. Claire describes the main reward of her job: 'It sounds like a cliché, but helping them, the child and family, and making a difference to them. Being able to do that bit extra, to make a difference to the family.'

A part of working with and supporting families involves staff gaining some insight into the reality of their everyday lives and using this knowledge to improve the support that is provided. For example, one of the healthcare support workers from Clinovia describes the juggling which she sees parents engaging in: 'When [name] is not at school, Mum's there with him, but she's also got the other children with her, so she's got responsibility for him, and them, and she's got to be with him all the time. So it's difficult.' The Clinovia nurse co-ordinators and Claire explain that the insight that they have into families' needs sometimes means that they can assist them to ask for assistance. The nurse co-ordinators comment: 'Sometimes we can see things slightly differently from the agencies that come in. A health visitor can come in and spend an hour talking to the Mum and then go away again, and depending on what day of the week it is, and how they're feeling, they get a different picture from us, because we're there so regularly.' This knowledge of families' needs that staff who work regularly with them develop also means that, at times, they can add their voice to families' requests for assistance. As the nurse co-ordinators explain, their knowledge of health and social care systems sometimes enables them to make requests in a way that is likely to produce a result. They describe how they 'might be able to articulate things differently than the family can. They might just be saying "Why aren't we getting this?" and we might be able to say, "Actually they need this because..."' Claire also identifies that staff who work closely with families may also be able to recommend additional sources or forms of assistance to them or provide them with information to assist them in decision-making. For example, she describes working with a family which was planning housing adaptations for their child, and suggesting that they should consider how things will change over the years as the child grows older as well as taking into account his current needs, because they will not constantly want to make adaptations to their house. However, Claire stresses that although staff can give advice or information, no one except the family can make decisions for themselves and their child: 'You can make suggestions, but eventually you have to say, "Well I think this, but I'm not going to be doing it, you are." You do have to try and see it from their perspective.'

As well as assisting parents to access support, understanding the situation in which they are placed involves listening to them. As well as listening to parents about matters which pertain to their child's care, one of the Clinovia healthcare support workers explains that supporting parents can include being available to provide contact with the outside world if they are unable to leave their home a great deal, 'One of the rewards is being able to listen to parents, because you are actually helping that parent. They may not have seen anybody all day, they might not have anyone else to offload to, and they need to talk to you about anything and everything.'

Working closely with families can be rewarding because of the relationship that staff develop with them. The nurse co-ordinators from Clinovia explain: 'You're not there for just a few weeks, you're there for a long period of time. They get to know you. You build up a relationship.' Although this can be rewarding, the level of involvement it requires can also be very demanding, as Sue describes: 'You're personally involved, you're there in the home, you don't just see the problems the family are having with that child, you see all the other problems, and you end up being Marjorie Proops really to the whole family. You end up sitting listening to the teenager who's having a bad time, and the grandparents, and you then realise the impact it has on them.'

In addition, working closely with families requires staff to develop relationships that work well for each individual family, which provide support, but achieve the right level of involvement for families and staff. One of the Clinovia staff describes the challenge: 'Finding the balance of how you're involved, working in a very intimate and very close way with the family, you become part of the furniture. In a way that great because it gives you the opportunity to really do your job in a very creative way, but also you have to be wary, when it crosses the line of how involved you get.' This is a very fine balance to achieve, and boundaries between families and staff can become problematic. Sue describes the importance, but complexity, of not overstepping professional boundaries and how, 'you do get drawn in, and it's a question of when do you overstep the professional boundaries with the family that would actually compromise you as a professional'. Similarly, in residential settings the relationship that has to develop to facilitate parents feeling welcome, involved and enabling them to maintain ownership of their child's care makes the line between appropriate and excessive involvement very narrow. Mary explains: 'Because the children are living here it's very easy to cross boundaries and get too involved. I think most of the staff have gone through one occasion when they have overstepped the boundaries to their detriment. I think we've all done it. It's almost impossible not to. You're here in a professional capacity, and they want to talk to you as a friend, and then you get involved with things that you don't want to be involved in and give opinions on, and it's very hard to step back from that.' Kate adds: 'You have to...it's as if you have to be burned, I've been here six years and it happened to me when I was first here, in the first year. It is very hard. Very, very hard. I find, overall, and I've always said it, that's what I find the most difficult thing here.'

This need to achieve the right balance of involvement is necessary for the well-being of staff and families, as Mary explains: 'What we try and put over is that you can't cross professional boundaries because, if that child dies, are you going to keep in touch with that family and give them the same level of input you're giving them now? And the answer is, no, because there are going to be other children coming through the door that you're going to be caring for and giving that support to. Or, are you going to offer them the same when they move on? Again you're not, because however much you think you will, you won't. So they will actually lose a friend, or a lot of friends at a time when they need support.' Sue adds: 'One of the big problems is that if a family does get very attached to one nurse and that nurse has to go, for whatever reason, then the family is totally devastated. Ideally, you need two or three nurses who know the family really well to prevent that happening. We don't want too many because the child needs consistency, not multiple carers. So it's the balance between enough but not too many, and also protecting staff, and by so doing also protecting the families.'

Equally, where staff are providing long-term, day-to-day support for children and families they need to get on well enough with the child and family for this to work as Clinovia's lead nurse explains: 'You have to get on with the family. On a ward you are with them for a limited time. In Clinovia it's not just for a week or two, and staff are with them at all times.' This means that individuals have to be able to negotiate a relationship that will work for them, and that staff and managers may have to accept that sometimes a member of staff may not be suitable to support a particular child. Tania explains: 'Families sometimes don't get on with a carer and they can change and they know that. It's OK, if they just don't get on. A few families have done that and it's not a problem.' One of the Clinovia nurse co-ordinators explains: 'They might be a brilliant carer, but, in a particular package with a parent…it doesn't work. It's a very fine balance, and we do sometimes move people around. It doesn't happen very often, but, you know they're perfectly safe, perfectly competent, but there's something about their personalities. Either they clash, or they get on too well.'

As well as these general principles, in order to support children and their families effectively, the relationship between staff and family has to be right for the individual family. Although some families like to have a degree of involvement with the staff who assist them, others prefer to maintain a distance, as Tania describes: 'We have a relationship with all the families, and every one is different. Some families will just run out as you arrive. They just want respite so they can go out. Some say, "I have three hours and I'm out of the door," and they use their respite really well. Other families depend on you for everything.' Sue also comments on the need to be able to work in different ways and in different relationships with each family, and to 'recognise when a family has had enough and doesn't even want to talk to you. Some families don't want to talk to you, and some nurses have said they've been let into the house but no one wants to talk to them, and I've had to say that actually that mother is exhausted and is having someone come into her house every night and she's got to make polite conversation for 20 minutes.'

This quest for the right level of involvement and compatibility between the child, family and staff includes consideration of the precise role which the person is fulfilling and how closely they are working with the family. For example, Sue explains that whether a member of staff works well with a family may depend upon whether they work alone with the child, or provide support when the family is present: 'The comments have been from some mothers: "That nurse, she is absolutely brilliant, the child likes her, the child's eyes light up when she comes into the house, I can't fault her on anything, but I just find I'm on tenterhooks when she's in my home." Whereas with another one "They're great with them, probably not as good as the other one, but I get on better with her, I'm more relaxed."'

Despite the need to negotiate the right level of involvement with the child, the family, and the right staff for the right circumstances, staff almost inevitably develop a degree of attachment to the child whom they support. This is a part of the reward of getting to know them, but means that, as Tania explains, when a child's condition deteriorates, or when a child dies, it is very hard for staff. 'Obviously you're not supposed to get too involved, but you can't remain detached, you wouldn't be human if you did that. You have to get involved.'

Respecting Parents

Working closely with children and their families requires staff to negotiate their precise roles, responsibilities and level of involvement with the child and the family. This negotiation is based around the principle that although parents may receive assistance to care for their child, the child remains theirs and, except in exceptional circumstances, decision-making remains with the child and their parents. One of the challenges of working with children in residential settings, in particular when they are expected to be there for some time, can be enabling and encouraging parents to retain this parenting role. Val explains the Griffin House philosophy:

'Although the children are "in care" they are still a part of their own families. Families therefore come and care for their children with our staff supporting them if they so wish, for example bath them, put them to bed, cook their meals. Alternatively, if the parents just want to enjoy time with their children we will do the personal care, cooking, and so on. They come along with us for day trips or just chill with their children watching TV. In this way the parent does not feel that they have "lost" their child to the care sector. We very much believe that just because a child can no longer live with their families either in the long or short term, for whatever reason, they still belong to the family and should have regular family time like all other children. Any other siblings are obviously welcome too.'

The situation differs in many ways when support is provided in the family home, but negotiating roles and making sure that staff assist and support families in a way that does not detract from the parent's ownership of their child remains crucial. For example, the nurse co-ordinators from Clinovia explain: 'That's one of the things that parents often say, you know, "I don't want to feel pushed out, I don't want to feel that I can't do his feed, or change him or bath him, or whatever." You don't always need two people doing the care, but you do need two around.' In this situation, negotiating on a day-to-day and even minute-by-minute basis, how the work of caring for a child will be divided so that parents have meaningful assistance without feeling that their child is no longer their own is a skill which staff must develop. The nurse co-ordinators add: 'Sometimes within a day who is the first or second person changes constantly. Mum might go upstairs, if she's doing a course, to do some study, and so then the carer is number one and calls for Mum if necessary, and then Mum comes down and gives him lunch or whatever, so the carer becomes number two, so it's this constant shifting of roles.'

Staff describe working with children and families in a respectful and non-judgemental way as vital, including respecting their childcare practices and choices. One of the Clinovia healthcare support workers notes, 'parents all do things differently. We all parent our children differently.' The Clinovia nurse co-ordinators also explain that, for families, having other people involved in their child's care means that their lives and decisions are visible to a third party in a way which other families' are not. In addition one of them commented: 'I think families often do feel judged, and we have to be constantly aware that we don't judge.'

Although a part of working with children and their families is working in a way that respects the family's values and priorities, this may occasionally present professionals with dilemmas. One of the nurse co-ordinators from Clinovia recounts a situation with one of the young people whose care she co-ordinates: 'A young lady who has very poor swallow, and the advice from the dietician is she should have no fluids whatsoever and only tasters of food. But when she is with her family she has anything she likes to eat and she drinks. And she aspirates and she gets infections. My personal point of view is that's not OK, but from their point of view, and from her point of view, she wants to take that risk. It's a very difficult one.' She goes on to explain: 'She can't do it herself, she can't pick up the drink and drink it herself, which she would do, if she could. But from my point of view, and Clinovia's, we don't do it, but even that, some staff would say, have we got the right, to say she can't make that choice? Because if she could physically do it herself she would. Are we denying her rights?'

This type of situation can be difficult for staff, both because of differences in their personal beliefs and values and those of children and their families, and because of contrasts between the rules or policies of the organisation or company that they work for and parents' ways of working. One of Clinovia's healthcare support workers explains: 'We have rules and guidelines that we have to work by, and it makes it very difficult when parents are not happy with the way we do things, or they ask for things that we can't do.' Although she acknowledges that parents have the right to care for their child as they see best, the development of a mutually respectful relationship means that parents also have to understand that staff are required to work within the regulations of their employer. The nurse co-ordinators describe how such situations can be handled: 'It's all about communication, having very frank discussions with families about things that are very difficult, about what it's OK for us to do, and just sort of setting it out and being very open about it. Making clear we're not judging them, but what our boundaries are.'

The need to be non-judgemental about families' decisions includes not making judgements about families' decisions over whether or not to care for their child at home, as Mary explains: 'Every single family that you come across is different, and every child and family will have different challenges, different abilities to cope, and learn and care. Or they might not wish to, and it's respecting that. Not everyone is cut out to care for someone with the level of disability that some of these children have. I always think to myself "Could I do it, 24 hours a day, seven days a week?" And probably the answer is no, and I've been doing this for a long, long time. I have the physical skills and understand how to do it, but emotionally it's totally different. So we have to respect people. It's not just can they cope with a child in a buggy at three years old, but can they cope with the fact that the child is never going to be independent. It's a huge, huge commitment.'

Working in Someone Else's Home

A particular aspect of their work for many staff who support children and their families is that the family home is their workplace. The nurse co-ordinators from Clinovia identify that this means staff being privy to a range of family interactions and information that is very private and personal and how staff 'go behind closed doors. We are in the four walls of somebody's private home.' This means that staff have to be committed to being 'as discreet as we can'. They add that a skill required to work in someone else's home is 'knowing when to disappear, maybe say, "I'll just go and look in the folder" or "I'll just take the child into the garden and play for half an hour" or whatever.' Although all the staff who work in the home setting describe the importance of being as non-intrusive as possible, as the nurse co-ordinators identify, this is not always easy and not all houses can comfortably accommodate extra people: 'The trouble is, these houses are not designed for having carers in them and they are tiny modern houses, with thin walls, and one reception room and a small garden, and there's a limit as to how far you can physically go away from the family.'

Working in the family home can mean that staff are an intrusion, albeit a necessary one, for families. This juxtaposition of being both a help and a hindrance to families is one which staff have to be able to understand and incorporate into their working relationships. One of the healthcare support workers from Clinovia explains: 'I think for me it's going into a family set-up and trying to think "How would I feel if I had someone coming in every night".' Sue adds: 'I think they do find, the parents, if they have big packages of care, and lots of people going in, they really do find it hard, someone going in all the time. It is just such an intrusion. How would you feel if you had someone in your house the whole time? How would you sleep at night knowing there was someone in the next room? You're there to give them a break, and some parents will say that it is wonderful and relaxing to know someone's there. But other parents will say, "I'm just sensitive to every little noise, if they go to the toilet in the night, if they go downstairs to make a drink, I hear it." Every family's different and every house is different. Some houses enable families to place some distance between them and staff, especially at night, but some do not.'

The intrusion that care staff constitute for families has to be taken in the context of them often being inundated with a range of other professional visitors to their home. In addition, all the staff who will provide them with support need to undertake a period of orientation and training related to the care that their child requires, and this intermittently adds a further person to the household. Clinovia's nurse co-ordinators describe how 'if a member of staff needs training, you might have to have two members of staff in there when you only need one, because someone's training them. And it might be that Mum actually wants to do the bath in the morning and change the trache tapes, but someone needs that experience, so we say "Is it alright if we do that in the afternoon or evening, so that this person can practise changing trache tapes?" Or Mum can change a trache tube in a few seconds, on her own, standing on her head, but actually this carer needs that experience, so it is going to be a bit longer and take a bit more time and might not be so slick as if she'd done it. Every so often, you can tell, people are getting fed up and sometimes again just a discussion about you know why we have to do this, we have to train the staff, this person can't be left on their own until they've had enough experience of this situation, so the sooner we get it done so that they can be up and running and a support to you, not a hindrance, which they can be at the training stage.'

Sue explains how this need to balance assistance and intrusion means, 'When we look at care packages for families it is a big balancing act. Families will often say, "I want 24-hour care", and I would always say, "Think very carefully about that, because it's actually very hard having someone in your home all the time." We review it on a regular basis, but have learnt from experience with other families that it is just so unbearable sometimes. It isn't any problem with the nurses themselves, it is just having a visitor for 24 hours a day, seven days a week. You're almost on your best behaviour all the time.' Sue describes what this means when making decisions about how much support a family requires: 'We tried and balanced it between how tired the mother was, how stressful it was looking after the child, but how stressful would it be having someone there all day, and look at the balance between it all for the families, and then review it regularly so that we would have the right level that would make Mum not too tired with having to do all the care, but would also mean she would have enough time on her own.'

In addition to balancing the intrusion and support for families, for staff, providing support in the family home means that someone else's house is their workplace. This contrasts with many other work circumstances where the workplace is a shared area for all employees, none of whom own it, and none of whom live there. As one of Clinovia's healthcare support workers notes, this means that there are considerations which when one is working in any other environment would not be an issue. These include practicalities, for example how far the employees' needs should be allowed to affect the family's environment and needs, even down to, 'thinking should I flush the toilet at night'. It also means that the atmosphere of the 'workplace' and the rules which govern it depend to a great extent on the individual family and will vary. Staff who work with more than one family must therefore be able to constantly adapt their working practices to the 'house rules' of the family whose home they are in. Although the need to work within the rules of the household is a part of respecting families, one healthcare support worker describes how, if the 'house rules' of the family make carers feel uncomfortable, this can have a negative effect on their work. She contrasts two family homes: 'In one home, if there's something wrong with the child, I…of course I worry, but about the child, not other things.' In contrast, in another home concern over everything around the child being precisely in accordance with the family's requirements can almost supersede her concerns for the well-being of the child himself: 'One family, I think, "Now, will they think I've used too many wipes?" It's ridiculous. There is one package where you are much more on edge.'

Specialist Skills and Knowledge

One of the rewards of working with children with complex and continuing health needs and their families that many staff comment upon is the variety and constant learning which it involves, as Mary describes: 'Every day is a learning curve…every child who comes through the door is always different, a different child with different problems that you've got to try and solve, things you have to learn with that child.' However, this can also present challenges for staff. As one of the Clinovia healthcare support workers explains: 'Every day is different. Sometimes, you don't want to expect anything, sometimes you would like to just go in and have the same day, but you don't.'

Developing the skills and knowledge required to care for children with complex and continuing health needs is also both rewarding and challenging. Healthcare support workers who are involved in this type of work often take on roles and develop skills and knowledge which exceed that of other staff of their grade. One of the Clinovia staff explains, 'when people say you're a carer, really you're so much more than that'. Another comments, 'in many ways we do things that are more complex than what trained nurses do'. The level of skills and knowledge that staff have is often highlighted when they contrast their work in the community to how work is organised in the hospital setting. For example, one healthcare support worker comments: 'You're more like a trained nurse really. I found that on the ward. Things I can do on the community, a lot of the staff who had been there [hospital ward] for years didn't know; I had to show them, and I was just a nursing assistant. So it is quite specialised. In hospital all the ventilators are down in the paediatric intensive care unit. But a child in the community has them at home.'

One challenge in supporting children with complex and continuing health needs in the family home is that as well as the level of skills and knowledge required, staff are often working alone. Although they can contact the child's parents or a more senior member of staff, physically they are often alone, as Sue describes: 'You're having to make decisions on your own out there in the community. In my previous job we took home a very, very unstable neonate with a tracheostomy. It was actually a huge responsibility. The baby had had respiratory arrests prior to coming home and it was quite a scary job at times, at two o'clock in the morning, when their breathing goes off a bit: when do you call the family and worry them, you've got no one to call and ask if they will come and have a look, and in an emergency your extra pair of hands are the parents, who are absolutely petrified when it happens, even though they've been trained. So actually you have to deal with it. In one instance we had to deal with a mother who was panicking, a father who was passing out, and the child going blue.'

This level of responsibility can seem daunting for staff, particularly at the outset, and for those who are not used to this type of work. A Clinovia healthcare support worker explains how she felt when, despite many years of experience in care work (mostly within the learning disabilities field), she first moved into complex care and supported a child who required assisted ventilation: 'I thought "My God, what have I done." I was a nervous wreck all the way through the first shift, by the time I got home, I was just mentally exhausted.' The child's medical and technical needs are often the major source of concern for new staff, as one Clinovia healthcare support worker clarifies: 'The difference is just the machinery. That's something that I'm not used to, alarms and lights, and you think, "What does that mean?"'

Although the medical and technical side of care may be the easier thing to describe as requiring expertise, and possibly the more acutely worrying for new staff, staff who work with children and their families also highlight the importance of developing their knowledge and understanding of the child, and of seeing beyond the machinery to the person. Val explains: 'Our belief is that Griffin Care can provide the training and ensure the quality of provision but we can't put into some one a love of children and empathy towards families. I say to the staff that I recruit their hearts – twee I know but true.'

As well as the level of responsibility that they take for day-to-day decision-making, staff can be isolated from direct support from colleagues. For instance, Sue describes how, 'you might have had a bad night: maybe Mum gave you a hard time, Dad was a bit funny, the child was unwell in the middle of the night, and there's nobody to sound off to. No one to provide the reassurance that its not you, it's just everyone having a bad night. You just go home.' Although the organisations that provide home care universally have regular meetings and encourage staff to contact each other for support, this is not immediately available in the way that it is in some other settings.

Organisational Issues

From a management perspective, staff felt it important that the support provided should enable families to manage their child's needs as best suits their lifestyle and priorities. Sue explains: 'The timing of the support that is offered is matched as far as possible to the family's needs, for example it may be in the evening, or during the day or at night. It's no good commissioners or whoever saying you can have three hours twice a week at this time, which is what they have done in the past. You need to be doing it when the families need it.' The Clinovia nurse co-ordinators also identify the need to make the timing of support revolve around the family's needs and to enable families to make the best use of the hours which they are allocated: 'For example, one family, both parents are learning to drive, quite intensely, having two two-hour sessions each a week, and so we try and give as much of the care as we can around that.'

While services aim to be flexible, and to meet individual needs, achieving this depends on staff availability and on being able to slot the requests or needs of all the families around each other. For example, if all the families who draw on one staff pool want the same hours every day it is impossible to facilitate this. Although the importance of matching staff to families' needs is indisputable, achieving this with finite staff availability is, therefore, not always possible. In some instances, staff availability means that families cannot access the support that they need, even when this is agreed as necessary. Sue explains that one frustration for families is, 'they fight long and hard to get the hours they want or need, and then the primary care trust or commissioners are unable to meet them because they can't get the staff, and so they have these hours, but then find there aren't the staff to meet that need. That is common throughout the country, and that is very frustrating.' Sue explains that, organisationally, the process of obtaining staff to support a family and maintaining this support can be a challenge: 'You get a new referral in, and you then have to get the staff in to cover it. In an ideal world we would like to have a team always on standby and then we can meet a crisis, if a child is ill, or new referrals, but in the real world you can't do that. We do have bank staff. This is absolutely crucial; to have a supply of bank nurses that you can call in.' As Val explains: 'My own view is that the budgets given for both health and social care are too small and therefore there is not capacity left for developing innovative, flexible services that can meet the individual needs of families. Budgets can only fund traditional services, and the thresholds are for ever being tightened in an attempt not to overspend. In my previous job I was involved in funding residential placements, direct payments, and so forth along with health colleagues, and it was very frustrating when you knew that a family had a real and genuine need for a service but that either the service was not there or the budgets could not stretch to individualised support.'

Several staff describe the organisational or political elements of their work as being the most challenging or frustrating. The Clinovia nurse co-ordinators describe the frustration of seeing delays in children being enabled to live at home: 'Even now you see children staying in hospital so long before they get to go home. It takes a long time organising things to get them out.' Alongside this is the inclarity or injustice which staff sometimes see related to service provision. The nurse co-ordinators explain: 'It varies. For some it seems you go to the primary care trust or look for access to a different discipline, and you get it. For others, it's like you're fighting, fighting, fighting. There's a huge variation in the amount of support that individual families get. It really is very individual.' They also explain how divisions within service provision can create a further problem: 'There is a political dimension or frustration as well, because it depends how a care package is funded. What category they're funded for. A lot of our care packages are category ones, which are all health, and so then social services say "Nothing to do with us" and I've noticed, certainly in one of the care packages that I'm involved with, she's category one, and social services won't get involved even with what is a social need because everything is funded from health, so from their point of view, she has no social needs. That is *very* frustrating. Doesn't everyone have social needs?'

Claire also describes one of the major challenges of her work as being 'red tape'. The increase in the number of children with complex and continuing health needs who are cared for at home means that the procedures, policies and protocols associated with this have also increased. While this is well-intentioned, Claire explains that it can limit the options or flexibility of provision for children and families, with procedure, rather than individuals, becoming the focus. Claire comments that at one time, 'you would figure out what would work for a family, but now there is likely to be a protocol, or guideline, which it is expected you will follow'. This may not always be appropriate, and requires staff to be confident enough to challenge guidance and interpret this in light of individual children and families' needs.

Summary

Staff who work with children who have complex and continuing health needs and their families describe a variety of rewards and challenges in their work. The most overwhelming rewards come from getting to know the children, being able to communicate with them, and meeting their needs – not simply their medical or technical needs, but their needs as people. This includes staff being a part of the mechanism by which individual children are able to be cared for in the best place for them at any given time.

In addition to working with children, being able to work with and provide support for the whole family is seen as rewarding. This brings with it the challenge of developing relationships with families that are supportive, but providing support in a manner which families find helpful, rather than intrusive, that respect and respond to parents and children's choices while working within professional or employment requirements, and which do not overstep boundaries. When support is provided in the family home, this can present specific challenges related to managing the necessary intrusion which staff create for the family.

The amount of responsibility that staff who work with children and families carry is significant, and can mean them having to develop very specialist skills and knowledge. Although this can be challenging for staff, the importance of learning about and becoming skilled in aspects of care beyond the child's technical needs and focusing on supporting the child and family holistically is recognised as vital for the provision of high-quality care.

Some of the major problems that staff describe in their work are organisational or political elements of provision and the reality that, with finite resources, not all needs can be met adequately or as individual as staff would like them to be.

Although staff described some very specific rewards of their work, there was a feeling that it carries its own intrinsic rewards. As one of

Clinovia's healthcare support workers puts it: 'I suppose really everyone here's got it in their nature, and that's our job. I think this is one job where there is no way people can do this unless you have it in you. There's something else to it. There's a pull. I can't explain it. You're in a situation where you don't feel you can leave, because it's a people thing.'

Chapter 12

Conclusion

The experiences which the families who have contributed to this book describe have highlighted many issues. These include things that it is important for those who seek to provide support for them to appreciate, and matters which it would be beneficial for society as a whole to be aware of.

Seeing the Child

One of the most important aspects of enabling children with complex and continuing health needs to achieve a good quality of life is to see them first and foremost as themselves: individual children and young people. Although their health needs are often significant, the way in which services are organised and children's needs are met should keep people, not procedures or tasks, at the centre of provision.

The importance of providing facilities and services which enable children who have disabilities, including those with complex and continuing health needs, to enjoy the same opportunities as their peers is enshrined in national recommendations (DoH 2001a, 2004). However, there continues to be evidence that many children who have complex and continuing health needs encounter difficulty in enjoying the same opportunities and experiences as other children. Despite findings from previous studies (Action for Leisure and Contact a Family 2003; Noyes 2006) and national recommendations (DoH 2004) children and young people's opportunities to engage in play and leisure activities, social activities, and to develop relationships with their peers often remain limited. This may affect their learning, development and self esteem (Noyes 2006), and diminishes their opportunities to have fun and enjoy life in the way that other children take for granted.

The provision of suitable facilities for children who have complex and continuing health needs in many areas of life often continues to be very limited. The examples of good practice and provision that exist make it clear that everyday facilities can be made accessible and user-friendly for them and their families. A much wider improvement in such facilities would enhance many lives, enable children and their families to enjoy more time together, and mean that children could be included in a wider variety of everyday activities, with their families and peers. Improved facilities in healthcare settings, in particular, would improve the quality, dignity and humanity of encounters with professionals. This appears to be a logical development given the increasing numbers of children and young people who require such facilities and who will access healthcare premises on a frequent basis.

Despite the *National Service Framework for Children, Young People and Maternity Services* (DoH 2004) making explicit the need for children being listened to, and Noyes (2006) describing the importance of all children being enabled to communicate, there is some evidence that children are not always afforded this opportunity. If, as is sometimes the case, children are not given the chance to communicate, or to learn to develop their communication skills, they are unlikely to be able to have their opinions and preferences heard. In addition, there is evidence that some individuals do not appreciate that children who have complex and continuing health needs wish to communicate and can do so if others are willing to make the effort required to facilitate this. Where children have difficulty speaking, their parents are often the most knowledgeable about their way of communication and can frequently act as interpreters for their child. Although using the skills that parents have is invaluable, these should be used as a means for others to develop their skills in communicating with the child, and as a means of including children in conversations and decision-making, not as a substitute for, or an excuse to talk over them, or without them about matters that concern them.

For staff who seek to support children and their families, acknowledging and valuing children's rights and abilities and making the effort to enable them to enjoy these rights and to achieve their potential is vital. This may be time-consuming, but forms no less an important part of supporting them than performing technical or medical tasks. There are examples of individuals who place the child and their needs, rights and views centrally when providing support, and see this as an integral part of their work. Where this happens, more opportunities become available to children and they are enabled to develop new skills, to enjoy themselves more, to give more, and to have this recognised. The converse is also true: where others, and in particular those who are intended to support them, do not view children in this way, their opportunities, ability to enjoy their lives, develop skills, and contribute to peer relationships and society become limited.

As well as the way in which support is provided, the attitudes which children and their families encounter in society are a significant influence on the quality of their lives. These include the comments that individuals make and the inquisitive scrutiny to which some children are subjected. This type of behaviour may have far-reaching effects for children and their families, not only in terms of feelings, but in relation to the opportunities and activities that they feel able to access, and families being able to spend time together. A more respectful, tolerant, and less judgemental approach by all citizens would enhance the lives of many children and families. This includes awareness of the potential for hidden disabilities so that families can be with their children in public without the unnecessary additional stress of encountering uninformed and judgemental attitudes and behaviours.

When the provision of services and facilities is being debated, as well as the value that improved provision brings to the child, the benefits to society as a whole should be taken into account. Where provision enables children to enjoy a range of opportunities, their ability to participate in society and contribute becomes greater. The benefit of improved provision should therefore be seen in terms of improving opportunities for society as a whole to enjoy the company and contributions of all its members. In addition, where children are enabled to enjoy opportunities to meet other children, socialise, and play with them, the ignorance that can breed intrusive observation, thoughtlessness and misunderstanding may be reduced.

Parents

As other studies have identified (Contact a Family 2004; Kirk *et al.* 2005; Carnevale *et al.* 2006), having a child with complex and continuing health needs can be very demanding for their parents and affects almost every area of their lives. In addition to the daily workload occasioned, there is a significant emotional aspect to having a child with complex and continuing health needs, and the long-term and unrelenting nature of a child's needs can make being their mother or father exhausting. Although it is impossible for those who do not work from day to day with children with such needs to fully understand the workload of supporting them, having some insight and listening to parents, to their priorities, choices and preferences is vital in providing effective support. Keeping the people who are parents as well as their children central to provision is essential. Ascertaining and acing upon what will be helpful for parents, rather than focusing solely on how medical or technical problems can be addressed is necessary if support is to be as effective as possible and to enhance quality of life for the child and their family. An important part of this provision is appreciating that, as Carnevale *et al.* (2006) have described, despite the often unrelenting nature of providing for their needs, the child often brings pleasure and rewards to their parent's lives. The support provided should aim to maximise these aspects of parenting and the relationship and activities which parents can enjoy with their children.

To provide parents with effective support, staff must appreciate that while families may need assistance to care for their child, ownership of and expertise regarding the child rests with them. As other studies and policy documents indicate (DoH 2001b; Kirk *et al.* 2005) this, alongside their finely tuned and intuitive knowledge of the child, means that parents can often provide professionals with a highly reliable indication of the child's condition and needs. Their expertise spans knowledge of procedures, conditions, and their child's very individual and specific needs and responses to interventions, treatment and approaches to care. As well as having knowledge and expertise related to individual aspects of care, parents often constantly engage in very complex decision-making about the fine tuning of their child's care and interventions, which, for their own child, they are unique in managing.

Although respect for the skills and abilities that parents develop is vital, effective and supportive relationships between staff and families also require families to be able to seek advice and be given information when their knowledge is at its end. Parents' expertise in their child's needs and responses is not a reason for staff to relinquish responsibility or to fail to contribute from their own knowledge base. In particular, where children require new interventions, or have a change in their health status, it should not be assumed that parents have the knowledge, skills or confidence to manage or treat these changes. What is required is for all those involved in a child's life to respectfully combine their expertise, knowledge and skills. This requires true partnership working. However, this is not easy to achieve and it requires consistent effort and honesty on all sides. Neither is this type of partnership something that can be dictated in policy or practice recommendations. Although recommendations for working in partnership are an important step, for this to be achieved requires genuinely respectful attitudes and values to be developed and a real desire to share expertise so as to provide the best and most appropriate treatment, care and support for each child.

As previous studies have identified (Carnevale *et al.* 2006), some parents describe a loss of contact with family, friends or acquaintances, and loss of common ground with friends as a result of having a child who has complex and continuing health needs. While this is perhaps inevitable, given the demands of their lives, it is important to be aware of the isolation which parents may experience, and for the support offered to enable parents to retain contacts with friends and family where they wish to do so. In addition, many parents describe some value in support groups, or contact with families who are also caring for children with complex and continuing health needs. Although it must be the choice of individuals whether they see value in or wish to access such groups, professionals highlighting their availability can enable some families to gain important social and emotional support.

Despite changes in employment policy and recommendations on improving matters for parents in this respect (DoH 2004), in most cases, a child having complex and continuing health needs affects one or both of their parents' employment opportunities. Although a variety of benefits and allowances may be available to families, the process of finding out about and claiming benefits can be very difficult and time-consuming. Given the other demands on families' time, this may mean that families do not receive the financial support to which they are entitled. In addition to the loss of income that changes in employment status occasions, the costs associated with bringing up a child with complex and continuing health needs is significantly higher than the cost of bringing up a child who does not have this type of need. Thus, for many families, the financial consequences of their child having complex needs are significant.

Despite the rewards and pleasures that their child brings them, parents often describe feelings of loss in relation to their child's needs. These may include loss associated with the child's diagnosis, or may be associated with subsequent events, changes in condition, or changes in the family's lifestyle which the child's needs create. In some cases, the losses that parents experience are ongoing, so that they describe a state of chronic but ever-changing grief. The feelings that parents experience can also be complicated by a mixture of grief and relief being felt concurrently, for example where a diagnosis confirms a serious problem with long-term consequences, but puts an end to uncertainty. The range of feelings which parents describe throughout their children's lives illustrates the importance of avoiding assumptions about their child's condition, their responses to this, and the effect that this has on their emotional well-being.

Support at Home

Providing support for families is vital, and the family home is usually the optimum place for children to live. However, as previous studies have identified (O'Brien and Veneger 2002; Valkinier et al. 2002; Wang and Barnard 2004), having staff to support them in their home can be difficult for families. This problem is difficult to resolve, because however respectful and considerate a member of staff is, they are still an intrusion, albeit a necessary and in many respects welcome one, for many families. There is an extent to which the need for support at home and the ability to maintain the family's privacy are mutually exclusive. An important aspect of providing support is therefore for those organising and providing this to appreciate this juxtaposition, and to be prepared to work within it, minimising the intrusion that they necessarily create, affording families as much privacy as possible, not being offended if the family find their presence stressful, and being open about this problem. Families who receive support at home should have the opportunity to discuss the impact that this may have when negotiating care provision, and they should be able to make truly informed decisions over the type and amount of support they would prefer. The variation in the impact of having staff in the home is reported to have on families illustrates that what will be right for one set of circumstances and one family will not be right for another. As with all aspects of provision, discussion and respect for individual wishes and preferences is the key to providing the best form of support for each family.

Given the close working relationship between child, family and staff, organisational and administrative matters should be designed to enable families to be involved in the appointment of staff where they wish to be. Although it is unlikely that every family will be able to be precisely matched to staff who will be their ideal, and the degree of involvement which families will want in staffing issues will vary, that they are offered the opportunity for choice and involvement, and are aware of the implications of their choices, is important. In addition, the staff who provide the day-to-day support for children should be as consistent as possible, so that they have the opportunity to build relationships with them and their families.

Families

As well as working with the child and their parents, as Taylor *et al.* (2001) and Sharpe and Rossiter (2002) have identified, it has again been illustrated how a child having complex and continuing health needs can affect all the members of their family. In terms of provision of support, there are examples of organisations that clearly see the child as a part of the family, and their role as being to support the whole family, including siblings. Where this is the case, the way in which the family is supported is clearly improved. However, in other cases the way in which staff remits are designed seems to militate against family-focused provision, which may worsen, rather than improve, the way in which families can function and the impact of the child's needs on the family.

Organisationally, the support that is provided should see the child as a part of the unique structure of, and relationships within, each family. This means policies and regulations enabling the staff who provide day-to-day support to work with the entire family towards improving their quality of life. It may also require changes in beliefs about the remits of staff and provision, and allowing staff the autonomy to work with the family to determine the best way of providing support, with what activities they require assistance, and to focus on working practices that facilitate children being a part of, not excluded from, their families.

Seeing the child as a part of the family includes consideration being given to how families can be provided with assistance to enjoy time together, including taking holidays. The needs which children have may mean that organising their leisure activities and holidays will always require greater attention than is needed for other children. However, how support services and organisations can lessen this burden should be given some consideration. While staffing is one part of achieving this aim, equally, leisure and public services need to be set up to enable children who have complex and continuing health needs and their families to enjoy time together, and take up activities and opportunities as other families do.

Short-break Services

Although enabling the child and their family to enjoy time together is vital, families also need to have access to reliable short-break facilities, and planned support should include back-up options for unexpected events. Again, this has been noted previously and forms an integral part of the *National Service Framework for Children, Young People and Maternity Services* (DoH 2004). There is, nonetheless, evidence that the provision of such services still has inadequacies, with families having to wait for long periods for short break care, and provision being unreliable or available in name but not in practice. As the number of children with complex and continuing health needs increases, it seems that short-break services are not increasing to meet this need. Like all aspects of provision, ascertaining from families how short-break services may be organised to best suit their priorities and preferences, for example in-house or out-of-home care, and the length and timing of provision is important. The evidence that families have different preferences emphasises that there cannot be a 'one size fits all' approach to provision, or a blanket decision on what is best.

Relationships with Professionals

Children with complex and continuing health needs, and their parents, are likely to have a number of encounters with health and social care staff and services. The quality of the relationship that they develop with staff is very important to the quality of their experience and care, and can significantly add to or reduce the stress of being or having a child with complex and continuing health needs. Regardless of the medical or technical skills and knowledge that staff may need to manage the child's condition, a major factor in the quality of healthcare for families is relationships between them and staff being respectful and staff working with them in an open and honest manner. The quality of communication and information-giving that they experience is vital. Professionals recognising and respecting parent's ownership of their child, and seeing them and their child as individuals and part of a family is also essential for high-quality support.

Although a child being diagnosed as having a certain condition should not detract from them being seen as an individual, having a diagnosis or clarity over the extent of a child's problems has benefits. These can include clarity over what the problem is and how it is likely to be best managed, more specific information, and the potential for support becoming available. The way in which diagnostic processes are handled is very important for children and their families, including the manner in which they are spoken to and the quality of the supporting information that they are provided with. As well as diagnosis, information on their child's likely prognosis is important for them and their families. While there will frequently be some degree of uncertainty regarding their likely prognosis, children and their families having as much and as accurate information as possible is vital to assist them when planning and making decisions about their lives. Again, where there is uncertainty, honesty is important, but parents having all the available information on matters that will significantly affect their lives and those of their children is essential.

Education

Children with complex and continuing health needs should be afforded equal opportunities for education as other children. The ideal is that this should be provided in mainstream education environments, in a way which truly includes and values the child (DoH 2001a). Although some families report that accessing mainstream education has been a very positive experience, there are instances where this has not been the case. This may be related to the attitudes of staff at schools, practicalities related to provision, or whether the child will be truly included and enabled to participate in the range of school activities. The importance of inclusion being real, and not tokenistic, was clearly identified as an important consideration in achieving a high-quality education experience for children.

As Berry and Dawkins (2004) identify, a child's medical and technical needs, and the provision of support for these in schools, affects children's ability to attend school and to engage in a full range of learning experiences, peer interactions and opportunities. There is some evidence in their study that a lack of staff to support children's specific medical or technical needs may adversely affect their opportunities to engage in education. In addition, there is evidence of varying degrees of enthusiasm or confidence by schools in relation to enabling children who need additional medical or technical support to access after-school or weekend activities. Where efforts are made to facilitate children to engage in all the activities that they wish and are able to do, their opportunities to learn and interact with their peers are improved. Where children attend schools which take a wide catchment area, how they can be included in peer activities requires some thought. While some schools show flexibility and creativity in this area, for other children it may mean that their opportunities are limited. Individuals, but also organisations, should consider how children can be enabled to enjoy all the opportunities that their peers have and which they are able and want to participate in.

When a child reaches the age at which further education is appropriate for them, this can create additional challenges, as identified by Millar and Aitken (2005). This includes a provision for a transition to further education, in particular where children have been used to small classes and one-to-one support. There is evidence that providing an appropriate transition period can positively affect a young person's ability to achieve their potential in further education, and to gain confidence and independence. In addition, at policy level, consideration should be given to how assessment processes and funding issues may be developed so that an holistic view of individuals can be achieved to enable young people with complex and continuing health needs to engage in lifelong learning and develop and achieve their potential.

Staff who Support Children and their Families

The amount of responsibility which staff who work with children with complex and continuing health needs and their families carry is significant, and often means them having to develop very specialist skills and knowledge. Although this can be challenging for them, the importance of learning about and focusing on aspects of care beyond the child's technical needs, and supporting them and their families holistically, is recognised as essential by many staff. In many cases the day-to-day care that children with complex and continuing health needs require is provided by staff who are not registered nurses. Although this is often wholly appropriate, it does require them to develop specialist skills and take on responsibilities for which they should receive recognition. If quality staff, who are able to provide the high standard of holistic support that families value, are to be procured to assist the increasing population of children with complex and continuing health needs they must be valued and rewarded. While many staff who provide high-quality care recognise that the principal benefits of their work are the intrinsic rewards of working with children and their families, their contribution and skills should be recognised and rewarded if more staff are to be attracted to such work.

Although the focus of providing support should be humanistic, not technical, the training that is available for staff merits consideration. Although many organisations which provide care for children who have complex and continuing health needs also provide their staff with comprehensive and ongoing education and training (Hewitt-Taylor 2005), in some cases, especially where agency staff are predominantly used, there is little funded training available for staff. In many cases this means that families have to train agency staff in their child's care. While parents often have unrivalled knowledge of their child's condition and needs, how they can be provided with updates on their initial training on the practical aspects of their child's care is not always clear.

Values

The experiences of children with complex and continuing health needs and their families illustrate that there are many matters that require attention to enable them to enjoy quality of life. The most important and overwhelming theme is that individuals should be treated respectfully, and that their views should be sought, rather than assumptions being made about their needs, values, priorities or feelings. Those providing families with assistance need to be able to provide the person- and family-centred support that they value. Learning technical skills is likely to be much easier to facilitate than changes in attitudes and values, and staff recruitment processes should have this in mind.

Despite the continued recommendations and evidence to encourage individuals who support children with complex and continuing health needs to retain their focus on the child and family, to see individuals, not medical or technical needs, there is still evidence that this does not always occur. There is also evidence that there are staff who achieve a very high standard in this respect. One of the challenges of providing quality support for children and their families is that legislation, recommendations or policy cannot dictate attitudes and values. They can create an environment in which better facilities are provided, and in which it is easier for individual needs to be met, but they cannot change mind-sets. Equal attention needs to be paid to how this can be facilitated as well as how physical provision can be improved. Both are vital; however, unless the ways of thinking of some individuals can be changed, adherence to policy and recommendations is likely to be a low priority or tokenistic, or 'support' may be imposed on individuals and families in a 'one size fits all' approach rather than being individualised to take into account the diverse population which children with complex and continuing health needs, like all other children, represent. There are likely to be many insoluble problems for children and their families, and there may be aspects of provision that cannot be easily or swiftly improved. However, the mind-sets that individuals encounter are not dependent upon funding. Although altering unhelpful attitudes may be the most problematic aspect of change, it is achieving this which will truly improve the lives of children and their families.

The challenge to which society as a whole, and health, social and education professionals in particular, must rise is developing beliefs and values that truly place people, not procedures, at the centre of provision, and which seek to enhance lives not simply transfer technology and medical care to the home environment.

Glossary

Apnoea: a transient absence of breathing.

Apnoea monitor: a machine that detects breathing and sets off an alarm if breathing is absent for a pre-specified period of time.

Aspiration: (in the context described in this book) taking foreign matter into the lungs.

Assisted ventilation: the provision of some degree of mechanical assistance to breathe. The degree and type of assistance provided varies.

Atrial septal defect (ASD): an abnormal connection between the left and right atria in the heart.

Attention deficit hyperactivity disorder: a condition whose principle characteristics are children being hyperactive, demonstrating impulsivity and having difficulty in paying attention.

Autism/autistic spectrum disorder: autism is the most common condition in a group of disorders known as the autistic spectrum disorders (ASDs). It is characterised by a person having difficulty with social interaction, problems with communication, and unusual repetitive or severely limited activities and interests.

Bi-level/Bi-phasic positive airways pressure (BiPAP): a form of assisted ventilation in which breaths are initiated by the child, but support is given to help them to achieve a good lung expansion and to keep the lungs slightly inflated at the end of expiration. This reduces the workload of breathing.

Bradycardia: a slow heart rate.

Brainstem: the part of the brain composed of the midbrain, pons, and medulla oblongata. This area influences a range of functions, including cardiac and respiratory functions.

Bulbar palsy: results from impairment of function of the VIIth to XIIth cranial nerves. This can affect swallowing and other functions controlled by these nerves.

Cannula: a small tube which is inserted into a vein or artery.

Cannulate: to insert a cannula into.

Cerebral palsy: neurological disorders which result from faulty development of or damage to motor areas of the brain (the parts that control muscle movements) which permanently affects body movement and muscle co-ordination but which does not worsen over time.

Chronic lung disease of prematurity: the results of the effects of positive pressure ventilation and high oxygen concentration on a structurally and functionally immature lung.

Complete placenta previa: an abnormal implantation of the placenta at or near the internal opening of the uterine cervix.

Congenital central hypoventilation syndrome (CCHS): a disorder of the nervous system where the control of breathing is absent or impaired. In the severest form, the child does not breathe adequately when awake or when asleep. More typically, the child breathes adequately when awake but not when asleep.

Continuous positive airways pressure (CPAP): a form of assisted ventilation in which a constant pressure of gases is delivered to the lungs so that they remain slightly inflated at the end of expiration. This means that the workload of breathing is reduced.

Craniostenosis: malformation of the skull caused by premature closure of the cranial sutures. This can mean that head growth is inhibited and, in extreme cases, the development of the brain and sensory organs is hindered.

Cri-du-chat syndrome: a group of symptoms that result from chromosome 5 being incomplete.

CT scan: a sectional view of the body constructed by computerised tomography.

Direct payments: cash payments made in lieu of social service provisions to individuals who have been assessed as needing services.

Dysphagia: difficulty in swallowing.

Echocardiogram: the use of ultrasound to examine and measure the structure and functioning of the heart.

Electroencephalogram (EEG): a mechanism of detecting and recording the electrical activity of the brain by placing electrodes on the skull.

Endotracheal (ET) tube: a flexible plastic tube inserted via the mouth or nose into the trachea (the airway) in order to provide ventilation to the lungs.

Extubation: (in the context of this book) removal of an endotracheal tube.

Fundoplication: a surgical procedure in which the upper portion of the stomach is wrapped around the lower end of the oesophagus and sutured in place (a treatment for gastro-oesophageal reflux).

Gastrojejunostomy tube: a feeding tube placed via the stomach and duodenum, with the tip terminating in the jejunum. This allows gastric access and direct feeding into the jejunum.

Gastro-oesophageal reflux: backtracking of gastric contents into the oesophagus.

Gastrostomy/PEG: the formation of an opening through the abdominal wall into the stomach to allow feeding directly into the stomach. A gastrostomy feeding tube is placed directly in the stomach through the abdominal wall. When the procedure is performed using an endoscope it is referred to as a percutaneous endoscopic gastrostomy (PEG).

Haemodialysis: filtering and removal of excessive fluid and waste products from the body by pumping blood through a dialysis machine.

Hemiplegia: total or partial paralysis of one side of the body that results from disease of or injury to the motor centres of the brain.

High frequency oscillation ventilation (HFOV): a method of mechanical ventilation which uses very high respiratory rates and low tidal volumes.

Hypoplastic: an arrest in development in which an organ or part remains small or in an immature state.

Incubator: a closed cot system which provides a controlled environment for premature or sick babies.

Intensive care unit: a service which provides people with potentially recoverable diseases with more detailed observation and treatment than is generally available on standard wards and departments (DoH 1998).

Intrauterine growth retardation: when an unborn baby is at or below the tenth weight percentile for his or her age.

Intravenous drug administration: administration of a drug directly into a vein.

Intraventricular haemorrhage (IVH): bleeding into the ventricles of the brain. The extent of the haemorrhage, associated ventricular distension, and parenchymal involvement is the basis of the classification system which describes IVHs as grades 1–4 with 1 being the least and 4 the most severe.

Intubation: (in the context of this book) the insertion of an endotracheal tube into the airway to enable assisted ventilation to be provided.

Ketogenic diet: a diet supplying a large amount of fat and minimal amounts of carbohydrate and protein.

Kohlschutter syndrome: a rare syndrome which has as its characteristics epilepsy, yellow teeth, dementia.

Kyphosis: exaggerated outward curvature of the thoracic region of the spine causing a rounded upper back.

Long line: a fine catheter inserted into a vein in the arm or leg with the end of the line lying close to the heart.

Lumbar puncture: the insertion of a fine needle between the bones of the spinal column in the lumbar region into the space around the spinal cord (the subarachnoid space) to withdraw cerebrospinal fluid or inject drugs.

Microphthalmos: abnormal smallness of one or both eyes.

Nasogastric feeding: feeding directly into the stomach via a tube inserted through the nose.

Nasogastric tube: a tube which is passed through the nose, whose tip lies in the stomach.

Nebuliser: an atomiser that produces an extremely fine spray for deep penetration of the lung.

Necrotising enterocolitis: tissues in the intestine become inflamed and start to die.

Negative pressure assisted ventilation: a method of assisted ventilation in which pressure is applied outside the chest causing it to move upwards and outwards, and air to enter the lungs as it does in normal breathing.

Neo-natal: of, relating to, or affecting infants during the first month after birth.

Neo-natal intensive care unit (NICU): an intensive care unit for newborn babies.

Neurofibromatosis: genetic disorders of the nervous system that primarily affect the development and growth of nerve cell tissues and cause tumours to grow on nerves.

Neuronal migration disorder: a group of birth defects caused by the abnormal migration of neurons in the developing brain and nervous system.

Non-invasive positive pressure ventilation: provision of assisted ventilation using a cushioned mask that fits over the nose or over the nose and mouth.

Osteomyelitis: an infectious disease of bone.

Oxygen concentrator: a device that extracts oxygen from the air and provides this in concentrated form.

Oxygen saturation level: the percentage of red blood cells that are fully saturated (carrying their maximum capacity) of oxygen.

Oxygen saturation monitoring/pulse oximetry: a system that measures oxygen saturation level as a crude determination of whether oxygen supplementation is needed.

Oxygen therapy: administration of additional oxygen during respiration.

Paediatric intensive care unit (PICU): an intensive care unit usually admitting patients aged 0–16 years, but excluding special care baby units and neo-natal intensive care units.

Parenteral nutrition: nutrition which is administered outside the gastro-intestinal tract.

Patent ductus arteriosus: the persistence of a normal fetal structure between the left pulmonary artery and the descending aorta.

Peritoneal dialysis: filtering and removal of excessive fluid and waste products from the body via the peritoneal cavity.

Pneumothorax: a condition in which air or other gas is present in the pleural cavity.

Positive pressure ventilation: a form of assisted ventilation in which pressurised gases are forced into the lungs to make them expand.

Pulmonary stenosis: an abnormal narrowing of the orifice between the pulmonary artery and the right ventricle.

Respite care: short-term care that enables a family to take time off from the daily care of their child.

Retinopathy of prematurity: an occular disorder of premature infants.

Rett syndrome: a disorder that occurs as a result of arrested brain development.

Scoliosis: a lateral curvature of the spine.

Seizure: the result of sudden interruption or disruption to the electrical activity of the brain.

Septicaemia: invasion of the bloodstream by virulent micro-organisms (e.g. bacteria, viruses or fungi).

Sleep apnoea: a condition that causes transient cessation of breathing during sleep.

Special care baby unit: a unit which cares for babies requiring continuous monitoring of respiration or heart rate, receiving added oxygen, being tube fed, receiving phototherapy, or recovering from more specialist care (BLISS 2006).

Statement of special educational needs (usually referred to as a 'Statement'): sets out a child's needs and the help they should receive in education.

Suction: (in the context of this book) a procedure that is performed to remove secretions from the airway.

Total parenteral nutrition (TPN): an intravenous infusion that provides all the fluid and essential nutrients which a child needs.

Tracheostomy: an artificial opening into the trachea to establish and maintain a patent airway.

Umbilical arterial line (UAC): a cannula that is inserted into the artery of a baby's umbilical cord.

Umbilical venous line (UVC): a cannula that is inserted into the vein of a baby's umbilical cord.

Ventilator: a machine that is used to provide assisted ventilation.

Videofluroscopy: a radiological diagnostic tool for the assessment of swallowing disorders.

Vitiligo: a skin disorder manifested by smooth white spots on various parts of the body.

Useful Websites

CCHS Support Group: the CCHS Support Group offers information and telephone support on congenital central hypoventilation syndrome (www.ukselfhelp.info/cchs/).

Changing Places: the Changing Places Consortium has launched a campaign on behalf of people who cannot use standard accessible toilets (www.changing-places.org).

CHASE hospice care for children: a charitable trust that supports families with life-limited children throughout south-west London, Surrey and Sussex (www.chasecare.org.uk).

The Children's Trust Tadworth: a national charity that works with children who have multiple disabilities and complex health needs (www.thechildrenstrust.org.uk).

Clinovia Ltd: a home healthcare provider that supports strategic health authorities, primary care and NHS hospital trusts, social and educational organisations by providing tailored home healthcare services. One area that Clinovia specialises in is providing care to individuals with complex care needs (www.clinovia.co.uk).

Contact a Family: a UK-wide charity providing support, advice and information for families with disabled children (www.cafamily.org.uk).

Julia's House: a registered charity that provides care in the child's home and in Julia's House itself for life-limited and life-threatened children throughout Dorset (www.julias-house.org).

Premature Child: a website for parents and carers of children who were born prematurely (www.prematurechild.co.uk).

Proactive parents: a support and information group based in Basingstoke, UK, for parents and carers of children with disability, whatever the age or disability of the child (www.proactiveparents.org.uk).

St Margaret's School: is a purpose-built, residential non-maintained school for children and young people with profound and multiple learning difficulties and complex medical needs (www.thechildrenstrust.org.uk; click on the Services tab for a link to the school's page).

Scope: a disability organisation whose focus is people with cerebral palsy and whose aim is that disabled people achieve equality and are as valued and have the same human and civil rights as everyone else (www.scope.org.uk).

Special Kids in the UK: a charity for families who have a child of any age with special needs (www.specialkidsintheuk.org).

UK Children on Long Term Ventilation: a website intended for the benefit of families and health professionals involved in the care of children and adolescents who need long-term mechanical ventilation (www.longtermventilation.nhs.uk).

References

Action for Leisure and Contact a Family (2003) *Come on In!* Birmingham: Action for Leisure and Contact a Family.

Appierto, L. Cori, M. Binnchi, R. Onofri, A. *et al.* (2002) 'Home care for chronic respiratory failure in children: 15 years experience.' *Paediatric Anaesthesia 12*, 345–350.

Balling, K. and McCubbin, M. (2001) 'Hospitalized children with chronic illness: parental care giving needs and valuing parental expertise.' *Journal of Pediatric Nursing 16*, 110–119.

Barrett, D. (2007) *Michael's Website.* (Accessed on 16 July 2007 at: www.michaelrigaud.co.uk)

Berry, T. and Dawkins, B. (2004) *Don't Count Me Out.* London: MENCAP.

BLISS (2006) How BLISS Can Help. (Accessed on 16 August 2007 at: www.bliss.org.uk)

Boosfeld, B. and O'Toole, M. (2000) 'Technology dependent children: from hospital to home.' *Paediatric Nursing 12*, 20–22.

Brazier, M. (2006) *Critical Care Decisions in Fetal and Neonatal Medicine: Ethical Issues.* London: Nuffield Council for Bioethics.

Carnevale, F.A., Alexander, E., Davis. M., Renick, J. and Troini, R. (2006) 'Daily living with distress and enrichment: the moral experience of families with ventilator-assisted children at home.' *Pediatrics 117*, e48–60.

Contact a Family (2004) *Flexible Enough?* London: Contact a Family.

Department of Health (DoH) (1998) *National Service Framework for Paediatric Intensive Care.* London: Department of Health.

Department of Health (DoH) (2001a) *Valuing People.* London: Department of Health.

Department of Health (DoH) (2001b) *The Expert Patient.* London: Department of Health.

Department of Health (DoH) (2004) *National Service Framework for Children, Young People and Maternity Services: Disabled Children and Young People and those with Complex Health Needs.* London: Department of Health.

Dickinson, R. (2007) *Dickinson Girls.* (Accessed on 16 July 2007 at: www.dickinsongirls.co.uk)

Donaldson, L. (2003) 'Expert patients usher in a new era of opportunity for the NHS.' *British Medical Journal 326*, 1279–1280.

Glendinning, C. and Kirk, S. (2000) 'High tech care: high skilled parents.' *Paediatric Nursing 12*, 25–27.

Hewitt-Taylor, J. (2005) 'Education for Registered nurses who care for children with complex and continuing physiological needs.' *Nurse Education in Practice 5*, 243–251.

HMSO (1998) *Human Rights Act.* London: HMSO.

HMSO (2005) *Disability Discrimination Act.* London: HMSO.

Kirk, S., Glendinning. C. and Callery, P. (2005) 'Parent or nurse? The experience of being the parent of a technology dependent child.' *Journal of Advanced Nursing 51*, 456–464.

Landsman, G.H. (2005) 'Mothers and models of disability.' *Journal of Medical Humanities 26*, 121–139.

MacDonald, H. and Callery, P. (2004) 'Different meanings of respite: a study of parents, nurses and social workers caring for children with complex needs.' *Child: Care, Health and Development 30*, 279–288.

Millar, S. and Aitken, S. (2005) *FE and Complex Needs. Views of Children and Young People.* Edinburgh: University of Edinburgh, Communication Aids for Language and Learning Centre.

Neufeld, S.M., Query, B. and Drummond, J.E. (2001) 'Respite care users who have children with chronic conditions: are they getting a break?' *Journal of Pediatric Nursing 16*, 234–244.

Noyes, J. (2006) 'Health and quality of life of ventilator-dependent children.' *Journal of Advanced Nursing 56*, 392–403.

O'Brien, M.E. and Wegner, C.B. (2002) 'Rearing the child who is technology dependent: perceptions of parents and home care nurses.' *Journal of Specialist Pediatric Nursing 7*, 7–15.

Office for Standards in Education (OFSTED) (2004) *Special Education Needs and Disability: Towards Inclusive Schools.* HMI 2276, OFSTED. (Accessed on 4 February 2007 at: www.ofsted.gov.uk)

Olsen, R. and Maslin-Prothero, P. (2001) 'Dilemmas in the provision of own-home respite support for parents of young children with complex health care needs: evidence from an evaluation.' *Journal of Advanced Nursing 34*, 603–610.

Parker, G., Bhakta, P., Lovett, C., Olsen, R., Paisley, S., and Turner, D. (2006) 'Paediatric home care: a systematic reviews of randomized trials on costs and effectiveness.' *Journal of Health Service Research Policy 11*, 110–119.

Shared Care Network (2003) *Too Disabled to Care? Bristol: Shared Care Network.* (Accessed on 5 February 2007 at: www.sharedcarenetwork.org.uk)

Sharpe, D. and Rossiter, L. (2002) 'Siblings of children with a chronic illness: a meta-analysis.' *Journal of Pediatric Psychology 27*, 699–710.

Stalker, K., Carpenter, J., Phillips, R., Connors, C., MacDonald, C., Eyre, J., Noyes, J., Chaplin, S. and Place, M. (2003) *Care and Treatment? Supporting Children with Complex Needs in Healthcare Settings.* Brighton: Pavilion Publishing.

Taylor, J. (2000) 'Partnership in the community and hospital: a comparison.' *Paediatric Nursing 12*, 28–30.

Taylor, V., Fuggle, P. and Charman, T. (2001) 'Well sibling psychological adjustment to chronic physical disorder in a sibling: how important is maternal awareness of their illness attitudes and perceptions?' *Journal of Child Psychology and Psychiatry 42*, 953–962

Valkenier, B.J., Hayes, V.E. and McElheran, P.J. (2002) 'Mothers' perspectives of an in-home nursing respite service: coping and control.' *Canadian Journal of Nursing Research 34*, 87–109.

Wang, K.K. and Barnard, A. (2004) 'Technology dependent children and their families: a review.' *Journal of Advanced Nursing 45*, 36–46.

Young, E. and Young, A. (2007) *Siobhan Tanya Young.* (Accessed on 16 July 2007 at: www.freewebs.com/siobhantanya)

Subject Index

Author Index

Lightning Source UK Ltd.
Milton Keynes UK
02 March 2011

168546UK00001B/34/P